WITHDRAWN

ORAL CONTRACEPTIVES: PSYCHOLOGICAL AND PHYSIOLOGICAL EFFECTS

Papers by
David P. Rose, Ben H. Douglas, Henry A. Moses, Abelardo Fuertes-De La Haba, G. Di   Paola, A. Leonard Luhby, N.F. Goldsmith, C.G. Thin, Daniel R. Mishell, Douglas M. Saunders, Emilio Carbia, Joseph Song, Tiiu Csermely, D.C. Smith, Hiram W. Mendenhall, L. Aftergood, M.S. Fahim, J.N. Fortin, Lennart Juhlin, S.B. Kar et al.

MSS Information Corporation
655 Madison Avenue, New York, N. Y. 10021

Library of Congress Cataloging in Publication Data
Main entry under title:

Oral contraceptives.

   1. Oral contraceptives--Addresses, essays,
lectures. 2. Oral contraceptives--Psychological
aspects--Addresses, essays, lectures. I. Rose,
David P. [DNLM: 1. Contraceptives, Oral--Collected
works. 2. Contraceptives, Oral--Adverse effects--
Collected works. QV 177 063 1973]
[RG137.5.073]   615'.766   72-13692
ISBN 0-8422-7101-5

TABLE OF CONTENTS

CREDITS AND ACKNOWLEDGMENTS

Aftergood, L.; and R. B. Alfin-Slater, "Further Studies of the Effects of an Anovulatory Drug on Lipid Metabolism in the Rat," *Journal of Lipid Research*, 1971, 12:306-312.

Carbia, Emilio; Guillermo Rubio-Linares; Alberto Alvarado-Duran; and Mario Lopez-Llera, "Histologic Study of the Uterine Cervix during Oral Contraception with Ethynodiol Diacetate and Mestranol," *Obstetrics-Gynecology*, 1970, 35:381-388.

Csermely, Tiiu; Edward C. Hughes; and Laurence M. Demers, "Effect of Oral Contraceptives on Human Endometrium in Culture," *American Journal of Obstetrics and Gynecology*, 1971, 109:1066-1072.

De Paola, G.; M. Robin; and R. Nicholson, "Estrogen Therapy and Glucose Tolerance Test," *American Journal of Obstetrics and Gynecology*, 1970, 107:124-132.

Douglas, Ben H.; Richard P. Hull; and Herbert G. Langford, "Effect of an Oral Contraceptive Agent on Blood Pressure Response to Renin," *Proceedings of the Society for Experimental Biology and Medicine*, 1970, 133:1142-1144.

Fahim, M. S.; D. G. Hall; and T. Jones, "Effect of Ovarian Steroids on Hepatic Metabolism. II. Estrogens," *American Journal of Obstetrics and Gynecology*, 1971, 109:558-563.

Fortin, J. N.; E. D. Wittkower; J. Paiement; and L. Tetreault, "Side Effects of Oral Contraceptive Medication: A Psychosomatic Problem," *Canadian Psychiatric Association Journal*, 1972, 17:3-10.

Fuertes-De La Haba, Abelardo; Gloria Vega-De Rodriguez; and Ivan Pelegrina, "Carbohydrate Metabolism in Long-Term Oral Contraceptive Users," *Obstetrics-Gynecology*, 1971, 37:220-224.

Goldsmith, N. F.; N. Pace; J. P. Baumberger; and H. Ury, "Magnesium and Citrate during the Menstrual Cycle: Effect of an Oral Contraceptive on Serum Magnesium," *Fertility and Sterility*, 1970, 21:292-300.

Juhlin, Lennart; and Sture Liden, "Influence of Contraceptive Gestogen Pills on Sexual Behaviour and the Spread of Gonorrhoea," *British Journal of Venereal Disease*, 1969, 45:321-324.

Kar, S. B., "Individual Aspirations as Related to Early and Late Acceptance fo Contraception," *The Journal of Social Psychology*, 1971, 83:235-245.

Luhby, A. Leonard; Myron Brin; Myron Gordon; Patricia Davis; Maureen Murphy; and Herbert Spiegel, "Vitamin B_6 Metabolism in Users of Oral Contraceptive Agents. I. Abnormal Urinary Xanthurenic Acid Excretion and Its Correction by Pyridoxine,'. *The American Journal of Clinical Nutrition*, 1971, 24:684-693.

Mendenhall, Hiram W., "Effect of Oral Contraceptives on Serum Protein Concentrations," *American Journal of Obstetrics and Gynecology*, 1970, 106:750-753.

Mishell, Daniel R., Jr.; and William D. Odell, "Effect of Varying Dosages of Ethynodiol Diacetate upon Serum Luteinizing Hormone," *American Journal of Obstetrics and Gynecology*, 1971, 109:140-149.

Moses, Henry A.; Clinton Battle; and Dottie Watson, "The Effect of Enovid on the Binding of Thyroxine to Plasma Proteins *in Vitro*," *Journal of the National Medical Association*, 1970, 62:331-333.

Rose, David P.; and Isobel P. Braidman, "Excretion of Tryptophan Metabolites as Affected by Pregnancy, Contraceptive Steroids, and Steroid Hormones," *The American Journal of Clinical Nutrition*, 1971, 24:673-683.

Rose, David P.; and D. G. Cramp, "Reduction of Plasma Tyrosine by Oral Contraceptives and Oestrogens: A Possible Consequence of Tyrosine Amino-transferase Induction," *Clinica Chimica Acta*, 1970, 29:49-53.

Saunders, Douglas M.; Stewart L. Marcus; Brij B. Saxena; Carl G. Beling; and Elizabeth B. Connell, "Effect of Daily Administration of 0.5 mg. of Chlormadinone Acetate on Plasma Levels of Follicle-stimulating Hormone, Luteinizing Hormone, and Progesterone during the Menstrual Cycle," *Fertility and Sterility*, 1971, 22:332-344.

Smith, D. C.; W. B. Hunter; and L. R. Spadoni, "Alkaline Phosphatase Concentration in Cervical Mucus," *Fertility and Sterility*, 1970, 21:549-554.

Song, Joseph; Milton S. Mark; and Matthew P. Lawler, "Endometrial Changes in Women Receiving Oral Contraceptives," *American Journal of Obstetrics and Gynecology*, 1970, 107:717-728.

Thin, C. G., "The Effect of an Oral Contraceptive Agent on the Concentrations of Calcium and Magnesium in Plasma, Erythrocytes and Platelets in Women," *Annals of Clinical Research*, 1971, 3:103-106.

PREFACE

Among the psychological side effects of oral contraceptives discussed in this volume are psychosomatic reactions, individual aspirations relating to early and late acceptance of contraceptions, and the effects of the pill on sexual behavior and the spread of venereal diseases. Those psychological effects which are considered include the following: blood pressure, binding of tyroxine to plasma proteins *in vitro*, glucose tolerance and carbohydrate metabolism, histologic study of the uterine cervix during oral contraception, and endometrical changes in women using the pill.

This book is a companion volume to *Pathological Effects of Oral Contraceptives*, also published by MSS.

Effects of Oral Contraceptives on Various Physiological Systems

Excretion of tryptophan metabolites as affected by pregnancy, contraceptive steroids, and steroid hormones

David P. Rose, M.D., Ph.D., and Isobel P. Braidman, B.Sc.

The metabolic pathway by which L-tryptophan is converted to nicotinic acid ribonucleotide is subject to the influence of a variety of hormones. In this paper, particular attention will be paid to the effects of adrenocorticosteroids, the hormonal environment of pregnancy, estrogens, and androgens upon tryptophan metabolism, as they are reflected by the urinary excretion of intermediates along the tryptophan–nicotinic acid ribonucleotide pathway. The possible mechanisms involved will be discussed in relation to more recent studies carried out in the authors' laboratory.

Adrenocorticosteroids

Tryptophan oxygenase is the first, and almost certainly the rate-limiting enzyme of the tryptophan–nicotinic acid ribonucleotide pathway. Its induction by glucocorticoids has been extensively investigated since it was first described by Knox (1). A direct correlation between tryptophan oxygenase activity in human liver and the level of kynurenine in urine collected after an oral dose of tryptophan has been described by Altman and Greengard (2), and is to be discussed by Dr. Greengard in a later paper.

A further study (3) showed that the excretions of kynurenine, 3-hydroxykynurenine, xanthurenic acid, and 3-hydroxyanthranilic acid are all elevated following treatment with hydrocortisone. Figure 1 summarizes the results obtained from these experiments. Treatment with pyridoxine caused a reduction in the amounts of all four metabolites excreted after hydrocortisone injection to levels that were as low as, or lower than, those excreted without hydrocortisone induction of tryptophan oxygenase. This seems to indicate that the liver contains a surplus of hydroxykynureninase apoenzyme that may be activated if pyridoxal 5-phosphate coenzyme is made

available to it by the administration of vitamin B_6. These results also suggest that kynurenine 3-hydroxylase activity is adequate for the hydroxylation of the increased quantity of kynurenine that arises from the cortisol-induced increase in tryptophan oxygenase, provided that sufficient pyridoxal phosphate is available to ensure that 3-hydroxykynurenine does not accumulate, but is metabolized to 3-hydroxyanthranilic acid.

An alternative route for the metabolism of the kynurenine produced by the enhanced tryptophan oxygenase activity is removal of the alanine side chain to yield anthranilic acid. The kynureninase that catalyzes this step also requires pyridoxal phosphate, and so vitamin B_6 administration would presumably allow an increased turnover along this route. Under normal circumstances, the enzyme has been shown not to be fully activated in rat liver (4).

Pregnancy

Elevated urinary excretions of xanthurenic acid in human pregnancy, with a return to normal levels following treatment with vitamin B_6, were described independently by Sprince et al. (5) and Vandelli (6). These changes were thought to be due to a deficiency of vitamin B_6 brought about by the fetal requirements for the vitamin; support for this view was obtained by Wachstein et al. (7, 8), who showed that the plasma and leukocyte levels of pyridoxal phosphate are diminished in maternal blood at term. More recently, Hamfelt and Hahn (9) have re-

Supported by grants from the Medical Research Council of Great Britain and the Wellcome Trust, and National Institutes of Health Grant Ph-43-67-1344.

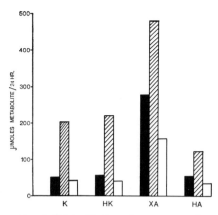

FIG. 1. Effect of hydrocortisone on tryptophan metabolism in a normal male subject. Excretions of kynurenine (K), 3-hydroxykynurenine (HK), xanthurenic acid (XA), and 3-hydroxyanthranilic acid (HA) following a 5-g L-tryptophan load are shown for: a control test (black columns); after 250 mg hydrocortisone by intramuscular injection given 5 hr before the tryptophan (cross-hatched columns); and after the hydrocortisone plus 50 mg pyridoxine on the evening before the test and again at the time of the steroid injection (open columns).

ported that early in pregnancy the excretion of xanthurenic acid is much higher for a given plasma pyridoxal phosphate level than it is for nonpregnant women with the same level of coenzyme. This indicates that the abnormal excretion of tryptophan metabolites in pregnancy is unlikely to be due solely to vitamin B_6 deficiency. In fact, previous workers had already suggested that tryptophan metabolism is modified by the altered hormonal environment of pregnancy (10).

Brown et al. (10) carried out a detailed study of tryptophan metabolism in the second or third trimesters of human pregnancy, and obtained data for the urinary excretion of both tryptophan metabolites and N^1-methyl-2-pyridone-5-carboxamide (2-pyridone), which is one of the two principal excretion products of nicotinic acid. Elevated levels of xanthurenic acid, 3-hydroxykynurenine, kynurenine, acetylkynurenine, and 2-pyridone were observed in urine collected after a 2-g oral dose of L-tryptophan. Treatment with pyridoxine produced a reduction in the excretion of most metabolites; although the

levels of 2-pyridone, kynurenine, 3-hydroxykynurenine, and xanthurenic acid remained above the normal range, the amount of vitamin given was less than that administered by Wachstein and Gudaitis, who obtained a complete reversion to within normal limits for xanthurenic acid excretion (11). Brown and his co-workers concluded that, in addition to vitamin B_6 deficiency, the hormonal changes of pregnancy alter tryptophan metabolism so that there is an enhanced capacity for the biosynthesis of nicotinic acid ribonucleotide from the amino acid. The report (12) that N^1-methylnicotinamide excretion is elevated in pregnancy is consistent with this view.

The published data would seem to indicate that at least two separate factors are responsible for the altered tryptophan metabolism of pregnancy: 1) towards term a true deficiency of vitamin B_6 develops that is due to the fetal demands for the vitamin with a transplacental loss, and 2) throughout pregnancy the endocrine changes are responsible for promoting the metabolism of tryptophan along the pathway leading to nicotinic acid ribonucleotide synthesis.

Estrogens and contraceptive steroids

The influence of female sex hormones upon tryptophan metabolism is not restricted to the gross changes of pregnancy, but is also apparent in the fluctuations that occur at different phases of the menstrual cycle. Elevated excretions of 3-hydroxykynurenine, xanthurenic acid, and 3-hydroxyanthranilic acid were found at the time of ovulation, when estrogenic activity reaches a peak, as compared with the levels immediately after menstruation (13). Further, a sex difference in the urinary excretion of metabolites following the administration of a tryptophan load has been described by several groups of workers. Michael et al. (14) reported that adult females excrete greater amounts of kynurenine, 3-hydroxykynurenine, xanthurenic acid, kynurenic acid, and 3-hydroxyanthranilic acid than adult males after a tryptophan load given in a dose of 100 mg/kg body wt, whereas Mainardi and Tenconi (15), and Rose (13) have also demonstrated a sex difference in tryptophan metabolism with

11

a standard 5-g dose of L-tryptophan. This sex difference was not evident when the loading dose was 2 g (16).

The role of estrogens in influencing the biosynthesis of nicotinic acid ribonucleotide was emphasized when Rose reported gross elevations of xanthurenic acid excretion by women taking estrogen–progestogen preparations for contraceptive purposes (17). These changes were observed only when urine was collected after a tryptophan load, and were reversed by the administration of large doses of pyridoxine. Further studies confirmed this observation, and showed that women using these contraceptive steroids excrete increased amounts of kynurenine, 3-hydroxykynurenine, 3-hydroxyanthranilic acid, kynurenic acid, and acetylkynurenine, as well as xanthurenic acid, in urine collected after a 5- or 2-g dose of L-tryptophan (18, 19). Treatment with pyridoxine reduced the urinary excretion of metabolites, including 3-hydroxyanthranilic acid, to normal limits. In addition to the changes in tryptophan metabolite levels women using Enovid-E (mestranol 0.1 mg, combined with norethynodrel 2.5 mg; Searle and Co.) were found to have elevated amounts of N^1-methylnicotinamide, but not 2-pyridone, both in urine collected without prior loading, and after a 2-g dose of tryptophan (20).

When they are given alone, estrogens produce a change in tryptophan metabolism identical to that which occurs in women taking the estrogen–progestogen type of oral contraceptives (Fig. 2), with the same response to large doses of pyridoxine (18, 21). When an adult male was given 0.1 mg ethinylestradiol daily, increased excretions of metabolites following a 5-g tryptophan load were obtained after treatment for 7 days. The excretion levels continued to rise throughout the 5 weeks of estrogen administration, and they rapidly returned to normal following cessation of treatment (18).

The progestogenic component of the estrogen-progestogen type of oral contraceptives does not appear to alter the urinary excretion of tryptophan metabolites. Figure 3 compares the excretions of 3-hydroxykynurenine, xanthurenic acid, and 3-hydroxyanthranilic acid by six young women who were not taking an oral contraceptive with those of five women who were using the progestational oral contraceptive megestrol acetate. This steroid is used both in combination with an estrogen (Delpregnin, megestrol acetate, and mestranol, Nova Industri A/S), and

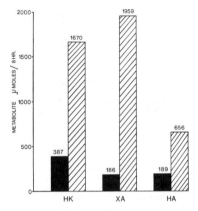

FIG. 2. Mean excretion of 3-hydroxykynurenine (HK), xanthurenic acid (XA) and 3-hydroxyanthranilic acid (HA) in 8 hr following a 5-g tryptophan load by 15 women taking an estrogen-progestogen preparation (cross-hatched columns), compared with 10 women of a similar age not taking a steroid preparation (black columns).

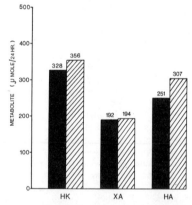

FIG. 3. Mean excretion of the same three metabolites shown in Fig. 2 by six women taking megestrol acetate (cross-hatched columns) and six control subjects (black columns). In this study urine was collected for 24 hr after the tryptophan load.

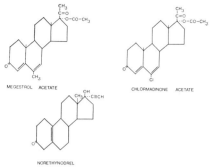

FIG. 4. Chemical structures of three pro-gestogens.

also alone, as a purely progestogenic form of contraceptive. It is structurally similar to progesterone in being a Δ^4-3-oxosteroid, and differs from chlormadinone acetate, the other progestational oral contraceptive, only in the substituent at position 6 of the steroid molecule (Fig. 4).

Norethynodrel, the progestogenic component of Enovid-E, has not been examined for its effect on tryptophan metabolism in man. However, this steroid may well alter the excretion of metabolites, for it is partly metabolized to estrogenic compounds in the body, and in fact, is chemically an estrane derivative: 17α-ethinyl-17β-hydroxy-estr-5(10)-en-3-one (Fig. 4).

Androgens

There is little published information on the effect of androgens upon tryptophan metabolism, although this is of importance in view of the changes seen in breast cancer. McGinty and Rose (22) have found that the administration of Mesterolone (1α-methyl-5α-androsterone-17β-ol-3-one, Schering Chemicals Ltd.) reduces the excretion of tryptophan metabolites after an oral dose of the amino acid. Prior treatment with this androgen also impaired the elevation of metabolite excretions that normally occurred after the induction of tryptophan oxygenase by hydrocortisone (Fig. 5).

Discussion

The precise site(s) of action of estrogens upon the tryptophan–nicotinic acid ribo-nucleotide pathway is not known with certainty. Rose (18) suggested that these hormones cause an increase in the activity of one or more of the enzymes concerned in this metabolic sequence, but that when the intake of the amino acid is considerably in excess of the normal dietary sources, as occurs in tryptophan loading studies, there is insufficient pyridoxal phosphate available to allow for the further metabolism of all of the tryptophan entering the pathway. This would explain why the N^1-methylnicotinamide excretion is elevated in urine collected without prior tryptophan administration, whereas the abnormal excretion of xanthurenic acid, 3-hydroxykynurenine, and kynurenine is only

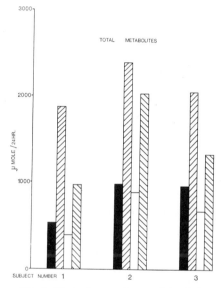

FIG. 5. Effect of an androgen of tryptophan metabolism in three normal adult male subjects. A control test was performed for which 5 g L-tryptophan was given at 2:00 PM (first column). Four days later 250 mg hydrocortisone succinate was given by intramuscular injection at 9:00 AM. An oral dose of tryptophan was given 5 hr later and urine collected for 24 hr (second column). Treatment with mesterolone, 20 mg orally three times daily, was given for 14 days. A third tryptophan test was then carried out (third column). Finally, after 3 more days of androgen treatment, another tryptophan test was carried out 5 hr after the injection of 250 mg hydrocortisone (fourth column). The values are the sums of K, HK, XA, and HA excretions.

demonstrable following a tryptophan load, and is corrected by treatment with large doses of pyridoxine.

If estrogens influence the biosynthesis of nicotinic acid ribonucleotide from L-tryptophan by producing an increase in the activity of a single enzyme, on theoretical grounds tryptophan oxygenase would seem the most likely to be concerned, as it is known to be hormone-inducible and it catalyzes the first, irreversible step on the metabolic pathway. This enzyme is increased in the liver of pregnant rats (23, 24), and also in female rats treated with a combination of mestranol, the 3-methyl ether of ethinylestradiol, and norethynodrel (D. P. Rose and R. R. Brown, unpublished observations) Recent work by the authors has substantiated the hypothesis proposed by one of us (25) that the effect of estrogens on tryptophan metabolism involves the induction of tryptophan oxygenase, and that this is mediated by way of the hypothalamo-pituitary-adrenal axis.

Pregnancy, in both rat (26) and man (27), results in a rise in the level of plasma 17-hydroxycorticosteroids. A similar increase occurs with estrogen treatment (28). Most of this increased steroid is protein-bound, and generally has been considered to be physiologically inert (29). However, Keller et al. (30) have shown that the rise in plasma corticosteroids brought about by estradiol benzoate administration is accompanied by an elevation in the activity of alanine aminotransferase, a cortisol-inducible enzyme, in rat liver. The enzyme was unaffected when the estrogen was given to adrenalectomized rats. The authors suggested that the protein-bound glucocorticoid is able to enter the hepatic cell by pinocytosis, and there dissociates from the binding globulin to yield the active free steroid, which is then responsible for induction of the enzyme.

Significant increases in alanine aminotransferase were obtained by Keller et al. (30) when estradiol benzoate was given by subcutaneous injection to adult male rats in a daily dose of 10 μg for 14 days. Figure 6 shows that an identical regime of estradiol benzoate administration produces a highly significant increase ($P < 0.001$) in the activity of tryptophan oxygenase in the livers of intact female rats, as compared with a

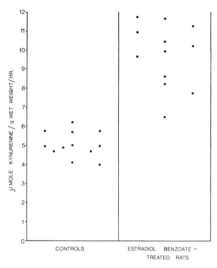

FIG. 6. Effect of estradiol benzoate on rat liver tryptophan oxygenase activity. These assays were performed in the presence of optimal amounts of heme. Control rats were injected with a volume of corn oil equal to that used as a vehicle for the estrogen.

control group injected with corn oil alone. Preliminary results indicate that the increase in tryptophan oxygenase activity does not occur in adrenalectomized animals.

The effect of estradiol on the adrenal secretion and plasma level of glucocorticoids is dose-dependent; large doses either fail to stimulate steroidogenesis (31) or actually cause inhibition (32). Consequently, the ability to demonstrate elevated tryptophan oxygenase activity in the liver of estrogen-treated rats depends upon the dose regimen employed. When intact female rats were treated with a massive 250-μg dose of estradiol benzoate daily for 14 days there was no increase in the enzyme level (Rose, D. P., and R. R. Brown, unpublished observations).

An alternate explanation for the abnormal tryptophan metabolism produced in the human by estrogen administration or pregnancy, but one which fails to explain the elevated N^1-methylnicotinamide excretion, is that estrogen sulfate esters, formed in the liver, inhibit kynureninase and kynurenine aminotransferase by competing with their

14

pyridoxal phosphate coenzyme for binding sites on the apoprotein. The effect of these steroid conjugates on the availability of pyridoxal phosphate for rat kynurenine aminotransferase is to be discussed by Dr. M. Mason in a later paper.

Estradiol disulfate has been shown recently to inhibit "hydroxykynurenine aminotransferase," the enzyme responsible for the production of xanthurenic acid from 3-hydroxykynurenine, in vitro, both in rat kidney and liver preparations (unpublished observations). If this inhibition takes place in vivo, and the very low effective concentrations suggest that it may, estrogen administration would not be expected to produce an elevated urinary excretion of xanthurenic acid. Although a high xanthurenic acid excretion is characteristic of the altered tryptophan metabolism of human pregnancy, the output of this metabolite is normal in the pregnant rat (35). There is, however, a raised kynurenine excretion, which is consistent with the known high tryptophan oxygenase activity. These findings may indicate a species difference in the behavior of kynurenine and hydroxykynurenine aminotransferase with respect to estrogen conjugates.

The clinical significance of the altered tryptophan metabolism by women using the combined estrogen–progestogen type of oral contraceptive is uncertain at the present time. However, one problem for which it may have etiological importance is depression, which is a well-recognized complication of this form of contraception.

There is considerable evidence that the level of brain 5-hydroxytryptamine is abnormally low in depressive illness (36), and three possible mechanisms exist for impaired synthesis of this neurohormone by women taking estrogen-containing oral contraceptives: 1) The amount of tryptophan available for 5-hydroxylation may be reduced, because it may be diverted into the tryptophan–nicotinic acid ribonucleotide pathway as a consequence of elevated tryptophan oxygenase activity. 2) The demand for pyridoxal phosphate coenzyme involved in the turnover of the tryptophan–nicotinic acid ribonucleotide pathway may be such that inadequate amounts are available for the decarboxylation of 5-hydroxytryptophan to yield 5-hydroxy-

tryptamine. 3) Estrogen conjugates may inhibit the decarboxylase by competing with pyridoxal phosphate for sites on the apoenzyme in the manner known to occur with a number of other enzymes (37).

These theoretical possibilities suggest that treatment with tryptophan or pyridoxine, or a combination of these two, may relieve depression due to oral contraceptives, although it must be pointed out that this occurs most frequently in those women using preparations with a high progestogen content (38), and the progestogens do not appear to modify vitamin B_6 function.

Our current concept of the changes in tryptophan metabolism that are brought about by pregnancy and estrogens, and perhaps by the abnormal hormonal environment of breast cancer, is summarized in Fig. 7, together with the possible ways in which these changes may produce diminished brain 5-hydroxytryptamine levels.

Summary

The effects of glucocorticoids, pregnancy, estrogens, contraceptive steroids, and androgens upon tryptophan metabolism in man are discussed.

Treatment with hydrocortisone produces an increase in the urinary excretion of kynurenine, 3-hydroxykynurenine, xanthurenic acid, and 3-hydroxyanthranilic acid, which is prevented by the simultaneous administration of large doses of vitamin B_6.

Pregnant women, those using estrogen-progestogen preparations for contraceptive purposes, and subjects receiving estrogens alone, all excrete elevated levels of these metabolites, although much larger quantities of xanthurenic acid are excreted than occur following single injections of hydrocortisone. The increased urinary output of N^1-methyl-nicotinamide in these situations is a reflection of the enhanced capacity for the biosynthesis of nicotinic acid ribonucleotide from L-tryptophan.

The progestogen megestrol acetate does not alter tryptophan metabolism when used alone for ovulation control.

Mesterolone, an androgenic steroid, reduces the urinary excretion of tryptophan metabolites, and impairs the response to hydrocortisone administration.

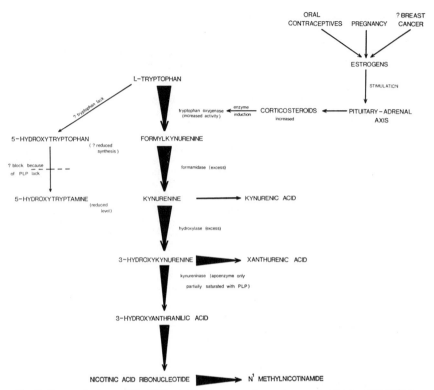

FIG. 7. Proposed scheme of the influence of estrogens and pregnancy on tryptophan metabolism.

The possible mechanisms by which pregnancy and estrogens modify tryptophan metabolism are discussed and, in the light of evidence obtained from animal experiments, it is concluded that estrogens cause an induction of tryptophan oxygenase that is mediated via the hypothalamo-pituitary-adrenal axis. Late in pregnancy, a true vitamin B₆ deficiency is superimposed upon the hormonal effects. 🌱

References

1. KNOX, W. E. Two mechanisms which increase in vivo the liver tryptophan peroxidase activity: specific enzyme adaptation and stimulation of the pituitary-adrenal system. *Brit. J. Exptl. Pathol.* 32: 462, 1951.
2. ALTMAN, K., AND O. GREENGARD. Correlation of kynurenine excretion with tryptophan pyrrolase levels in disease and after hydrocortisone induction. *J. Clin. Invest.* 45: 1527, 1966.
3. ROSE, D. P., AND F. MCGINTY. The influence of adrenocortical hormones and vitamins upon tryptophan metabolism in man. *Clin. Sci.* 35: 1, 1968.
4. ROSE, D. P., AND R. R. BROWN. The influence of sex and estrogens on liver kynureninase and kynurenine aminotransferase in the rat. *Biochim. Biophys. Acta* 184: 412, 1969.
5. SPRINCE, H., R. S. LOWY, C. E. FOLSOME AND J. S. BEHRMAN. Studies on the urinary excretion of "xanthurenic acid" during normal and abnormal pregnancy: a survey of the excretion of "xanthurenic acid" in normal nonpregnant, normal pregnant, pre-eclamptic, and eclamptic women. *Am. J. Obstet. Gynecol.* 62: 84, 1951.
6. VANDELLI, I. The use of vitamin B₆ (pyridoxine) for suppressing the elimination of xanthurenic acid in pregnant and non-pregnant women following the oral intake of a measured quantity of tryptophan. (Ital.) *Acta Vitaminol.* 5: 55, 1951.
7. WACHSTEIN, M., C. MOORE AND L. W. GRAFFEO. Pyridoxal phosphate (B₆-al-PO₄) levels of circulating leukocytes in maternal and cord blood. *Proc. Soc. Exptl. Biol. Med.* 96: 326, 1957.
8. WACHSTEIN, M., J. D. KELLNER AND J. M.

ORITZ. Pyridoxal phosphate in plasma and leukocytes of normal and pregnant subjects following B_6 load tests. *Proc. Soc. Exptl. Biol. Med.* 103: 350, 1960.

9. HAMFELT, A., AND L. HAHN. Pyridoxal phosphate concentration in plasma and tryptophan load test during pregnancy. *Clin. Chim. Acta* 25: 91, 1969.

10. BROWN, R. R., M. J. Thornton AND J. M. PRICE. The effect of vitamin supplementation on the urinary excretion of tryptophan metabolites by pregnant women. *J. Clin. Invest.* 40: 617, 1961.

11. WACHSTEIN, M., AND A. GUDAITIS. Disturbance of vitamin B_6 metabolism in pregnancy. III. The influence of various amounts of pyridoxine hydrochloride upon the abnormal tryptophane load test in pregnant women. *J. Lab. Clin. Med.* 42: 98, 1953.

12. HERNANDEZ, T. Tryptophan metabolite excretion in pregnancy after a tryptophan load test. *Federation Proc.* 23: 136, 1964.

13. ROSE, D. P. The influence of sex, age and breast cancer on tryptophan metabolism. *Clin. Chim. Acta* 18: 221, 1967.

14. MICHAEL, A. F., K. N. DRUMMOND, D. DOEDEN, J. A. ANDERSON AND R. A. GOOD. Tryptophan metabolism in man. *J. Clin. Invest.* 43: 1730, 1964.

15. MAINARDI, L., AND L. T. TENCONI. Contribution to the study of the tryptophan → nicotinic acid line metabolites in relation to sex. (Ital.). Acta Vitaminol. 18: 249, 1964.

16. PRICE, J. M., R. R. BROWN AND N. YESS. Testing the functional capacity of the tryptophan-niacin pathway in man by analysis of urinary metabolites. In: *Advances in Metabolic Disorders*, edited by R. Levine and R. Luft. New York: Academic, 1965, vol. 2, p. 159.

17. ROSE, D. P. Excretion of xanthurenic acid in the urine of women taking progestogen-oestrogen preparations. *Nature* 210: 196, 1966.

18. ROSE, D. P. The influence of oestrogens on tryphophan metabolism in man. *Clin. Sci.* 31: 265, 1966.

19. PRICE, J. M., M. J. THORNTON AND L. M. MUELLER. Tryptophan metabolism in women using steroid hormones for ovulation control. *Am. J. Clin. Nutr.* 20: 452, 1967.

20. ROSE, D. P., R. R. BROWN AND J. M. PRICE. Metabolism of tryptophan to nicotinic acid derivatives by women taking oestrogen-progestogen preparations. *Nature* 219: 1259, 1968.

21. BROWN, R. R., D. P. ROSE, J. M. PRICE AND H. WOLF. Tryptophan metabolism as affected by anovulatory agents. *Ann. N. Y. Acad. Sci.* 166: 44, 1969.

22. McGINTY, F., AND D. P. ROSE. Influence of

androgens upon tryptophan metabolism in man. *Life Sci.* 8: 1193, 1969.

23. AURICCHIO, S., N. RIGILLO AND R. DI TORO. Researches on the biosynthesis of nicotinic acid from tryptophan during pregnancy, the foetal and the neonatal periods. I. Tryptophan pyrrolase and 3-hydroxyanthranilic oxidase activity of the rat liver. (Ital.). *Minerva Pediat.* 12: 1463, 1960.

24. GREENGARD, P., H. J. KALINSKY AND T. J. MANNING. Tryptophan pyrrolase activity during pregnancy. *Biochim. Biophys. Acta* 156: 198, 1968.

25. ROSE, D. P. Oral contraceptives and depression. *Lancet* 2: 321, 1969.

26. HOET, J. J., G. PAGNI, E. EKKA AND G. C. SABA. In: *Hormonal Steroids*, edited by L. Martini and A. Pecile. New York: Academic, 1965, vol. 2, p. 341.

27. GEMZELL, C. A. Blood levels of 17-hydroxy-corticosteroids in normal pregnancy. *J. Clin. Endocrinol. Metab.* 13: 898, 1953.

28. WALLACE, E. Z., H. I. SILVERBERG AND A. C. CARTER. Effect of ethinyl estradiol on plasma 17-hydroxycorticosteroids, ACTH responsiveness and hydrocortisone clearance in man. *Proc. Soc. Exptl. Biol. Med.* 95: 805, 1957.

29. SLAUNWHITE, W. R., JR., AND A. A. SANDBERG. Transcortin: a corticosteroid-binding protein of plasma. *J. Clin. Invest.* 38: 384, 1959.

30. KELLER, N., U. I. RICHARDSON AND F. E. YATES. Protein binding and the biological activity of corticosteroids: *in vivo* induction of hepatic and pancreatic alanine amino-transferases by corticosteroids in normal and estrogen-treated rats. *Endocrinology* 84: 49, 1969.

31. D'ANGELO, S. A. Simultaneous effects of estradiol on TSH secretion and adrenocortical function in male and female rats. *Endocrinology* 82: 1035, 1968.

32. KITAY, J. I. Effects of estradiol on pituitary-adrenal function in male and female rats. *Endocrinology* 72: 947, 1963.

33. MAINARDI, L. Aspects of tryptophan metabolism during pregnancy in various species of animals. (Ital.) *Acta Vitaminol.* 3: 110, 1947.

34. CURZON, G. Tryptophan pyrrolase—a biochemical factor in depressive illness? *Brit. J. Psychiat.* 115: 1367, 1969.

35. MASON, M., J. FORD AND H. L. C. WU. Effects of steroid and nonsteroid metabolites on enzyme conformation and pyridoxal phosphate binding. *Ann. N. Y. Acad. Sci.* 166: 170, 1969.

36. GRANT, E. C. G., AND E. MEARS. Mental effects of oral contraceptives. *Lancet* 2: 945, 1967.

Discussion

I. P. Braidman: As an extension to the study of tryptophan oxygenase, described by Dr. Rose, we have now obtained some preliminary results for the activity of this enzyme and of alanine aminotransferase in adrenalectomized rats.

Our results confirm the observations by

Keller and co-workers (1) that the level of alanine aminotransferase as well as tryptophan oxygenase is elevated in the liver of intact female rats treated with 10 μg estradiol benzoate daily for 14 days. Results are expressed in millimoles of pyruvate produced per gram wet liver weight per hour, and the difference from the control is highly significant ($P < 0.001$).

We have summarized the data from experiments with control and estrogen-treated adrenalectomized rats and compared these with the situation in intact controls. There was no difference in the alanine aminotransferase activity among the three groups. However, the level in tryptophan oxygenase in the control adrenalectomized rats was significantly lower than in the intact controls ($P < 0.001$). Treatment with estradiol benzoate produced an apparent increase in tryptophan oxygenase activity as compared with controls after adrenalectomy ($0.5 < P < 0.1$), although the levels were still lower than those of the intact controls. We conclude from these results that the very high activities seen in estrogen-treated rats were a consequence of glucocorticoid induction.

An explanation for the higher level of tryptophan oxygenase activity in the estrogen-treated rats after adrenalectomy as compared with adrenalectomized controls may lie with the capacity of conjugated estrogens to stabilize cortisol-inducible enzymes. This has been reported for tyrosine aminotransferase (2) and it may be that the substantial decrease in tryptophan oxygenase activity observed in the control adrenalectomized rats is offset to a certain extent through a stabilization of the enzyme by estradiol benzoate.

R. A. Wapnir: Is there information on how much urinary tryptophan is excreted after load tests in estrogen-treated or untreated women?

D. P. Rose: In the normal subject Michael and his co-workers found, using a 100-mg/kg body wt dose of L-tryptophan, that there were just traces of the amino acid in the urine after the load. The amino acid has been fully metabolized somewhere, although clearly not in the metabolites that we determine under such conditions. I don't know of any data on the output of tryptophan in estrogen-treated women.

J. E. Leklem: In that respect, Dr. Rose, I would like to ask you why you chose a 2:00 PM time for administering your load of tryptophan?

D. P. Rose: Well, normally I do not. My regular time is 9:00 AM but in these hydrocortisone studies I wanted to allow for a period of induction after giving the hydrocortisone. So to

avoid coming in to the laboratory in the middle of the night to give the hydrocortisone, we set our study up so that we gave the hydrocortisone at 9:00 AM and then 5 hr later, at 2:00 PM, we gave the tryptophan load. This schedule was used only in this study.

F. Rosen: Is there any evidence that estradiol can induce an increase in the activity of either the kynurenine transaminase or kynureninase enzymes?

D. P. Rose: Yes, we found some data that surprise us a bit on the effect of a combination of mestranol and norethynodrel on kynureninase in rat liver and we did find there that this combination of steroids elevated the activity of kynureninase. This was distinct from what we found with the natural steroid, estradiol. Estradiol inhibited kynureninase activity in the male rat but not in the female rat. We observed a sex difference, and this has been reported previously by Dr. Mason; the male rat has a higher activity of kynureninase in the liver than the female rat. When we gave 20 μg estradiol daily for 28 days to the male rat, the activity of the enzyme came down to the female level. When we gave the hormone to female rats, either in that or in much larger doses, there was no further reduction but we did find this difference between the natural steroid and the synthetic steroid combination.

P. Swan: Does estrogen administration change the metabolism of sulfur amino acids? This would provide evidence as to whether or not estrogen interferes generally with B_6-requiring enzymes by interfering with pyridoxine metabolism.

D. P. Rose: I know of no in vivo studies of this type. Dr. Mason, I believe, included sulfur-metabolizing enzymes in the spectrum of enzymes that he studied, and did find that conjugates inhibit these enzymes in vitro. I am speaking off the cuff, but I think I am remembering it right.

B. Clark: Do cortisol conjugates also stabilize tryptophan pyrrolase?

D. P. Rose: We haven't done any studies on this.

H. Spiera: Do you have any information as to the minimal amount of cortisone necessary to increase excretion of kynurenine?

D. P. Rose: McGinty, who is working in Sheffield, did some studies on this that haven't been published. He got down to 50 mg hydrocortisone succinate, starting at 250 mg and then going down by small increments, doing the

18

studies at weekly intervals and always using a 5-g load of L-tryptophan. With 50 mg hydrocortisone succinate he thought that he had just about reached the minimum quantity that would produce a response, but this work is quite preliminary.

R. R. P. Warner: Is there a significant change in urinary metabolites excreted after oral load of L-tryptophan in normal human females during different times in the menstrual cycle?

D. P. Rose: Yes, there is. Two studies, one from Dr. Brown using a 2-g load, and one from our laboratory using a 5-g load. In both studies there was a difference, with higher excretions of metabolites at the time of ovulation (about the 13th day of the cycle) than when the loading test was done immediately after the menstrual cycle. Again, I think our data were more clear-cut than Dr. Brown's because we were giving a 5-g load and this load was better when endogenous variations of hormones are studied.

G. A. Abdel-Tawab: If the concentration of ethinylestradiol is decreased, say, to 0.05 mg/pill, do you think the tryptophan metabolism will be normal under such conditions?

D. P. Rose: With 0.05 mg of ethinylestradiol, the excretions are still grossly abnormal (*Clin. Sci.* 31: 265, 1966).

N. Narasimhachari: Have serotonin or 5-hydroxyindoleacetic acid levels been done on estradiol-treated subjects?

D. P. Rose: I do not think so. I have no data and have not seen any published data either.

R. A. Toseland: We have demonstrated how one can detect spontaneous, i.e., nonloaded, levels of 3-hydroxyanthranilic acid in a female patient before taking the oral contraceptive. The significance of this is that if the patient were taking salicylates they would appear well separated from 3-hydroxyanthranilic acid. This technique of thin-layer electrophoresis on cellulose avoids the problems of paper chromatography when the metabolites clash or migrate to the same place. The determination is much faster and the extraction of the metabolites from powdered cellulose is also much faster than from paper.

G. A. Abdel-Tawab: We investigated the interrelation between female sex hormones and tryptophan metabolism along the kynurenine pathway in different age groups of women after loading with 2 g tryptophan, with and without 120-mg vitamin B$_6$ supplementation. The following groups were studied:

Group I. Young nonpregnant women, ages 23 to 40 years, included the following subgroups: *Subgroup A:* Fourteen cases were studied in the preovulatory phase when the prevailing female sex hormones are natural estrogens. Urine collection was started on the 9th day of the menstrual cycle. *Subgroup B:* Eight cases were studied in the postovulatory phase, starting on the 23rd day of the menstrual cycle when both natural estrogens and progestogens are produced.

Group II. Young, nonpregnant women under the effect of synthetic hormones, started early in the menstrual cycle, included three subgroups: *Subgroup A:* Eighteen cases given ethinylestradiol (0.05 mg tablets) one tablet daily from the 5th day of the menstrual cycle for 2 weeks. *Subgroup B:* Ten cases were given norethisterone (5 mg tablets) one tablet daily from the 5th day of the menstrual cycle for 2 weeks. *Subgroup C:* Twenty-two cases were studied during oral contraception with 3 mg norethisterone acetate plus 0.05 mg ethinylestradiol (the oral contraceptive commonly used in the United Arab Republic under the trade name Gyn-Anovlar), one pill daily from the 5th day of the cycle for 21 days.

Group III. Nine cases were women in the postmenopausal age (ages between 47 and 60 years).

Group IV: Fourteen nonsmoker males aged 20 to 40 years, were chosen as controls. The controls, as well as the different groups of women, were compared with respect to their ability to metabolize the tryphophan load, with and without B$_6$ supplementation. Subtraction of the basal level of the urinary metabolites from the levels in either the posttryptophan or the posttryptophan–pyridoxine urines gives the response of each individual to the loading dose of L-tryptophan; that is, *yield I* and *yield II*, respectively, expressed as the quantity, in milligrams/24-hr urine, excreted in excess of the basal level.

The tryptophan loading schedule, as mentioned above, was started at the anticipated time of ovulation or just prior to the time of menstruation in *subgroups A, B,* and *C* of *Group II.*

1) The results showed that in young, nonpregnant women in the preovulatory phase under the effect of natural estrogens there was accumulation of some bladder carcinogens, mainly 3-hydroxykynurenine and 3-hydroxyanthranilic acid, as well as some other tryptophan metabolites that included o-aminohippuric acid, acetylkynurenine, and kynurenine. This suggests that the degradation of 3-hydroxyanthranilic acid to niacin was impaired. This inhibition was corrected by vitamin B$_6$ supplementation, indicating that the B_6-dependent quinolinic acid decarboxylase may be the enzyme that suffers inhibition in this group.

2) In young, nonpregnant women in the postovulatory phase under the effect of both naturally occurring estrogens and progestogens, the excretion level of different metabolites was about the same as or less than that of controls. This means that the excretion pattern was corrected by progesterone, which antagonized the effect of estrogens. After a loading dose of vitamin B_6, these women excreted more 4-pyridoxic acid than controls. This means that there was a decreased requirement for vitamin B_6 in the postovulatory phase.

3) In the postmenopausal women there was an accumulation to kynurenine, acetylkynurenine, and 3-hydroxykynurenine, and decreased production of anthranilic acid glucuronide and 3-hydroxyanthranilic acid, as well as decreased production of kynurenic acid and xanthurenic acid. This means that there was inhibition of the B_6-dependent kynureninase and transaminases. Pyridoxine supplementation partially corrected the inhibition, especially that of 3-hydroxykynurenine transaminase.

Thus, there was functional pyridoxine deficiency in young nonpregnant women in the preovulatory phase, as well as in the women in the postmenopausal age. This may be due to the hormonal pattern prevailing. If this is the case, then one would expect that suppression of the naturally occurring ovarian estrogens will alter the excretion pattern of young, nonpregnant women in the preovulatory phase to that of the controls with normal enzymic reactions along the kynurenine pathway. Indeed, this was the case. Thus, under the effect of ethinylestradiol alone, we got a normal pattern; kynurenic acid,

acetylkynurenine, kynurenine, xanthurenic acid, and 3-hydroxyanthranilic acid were less than the corresponding values of young, nonpregnant women in the preovulatory phase. Furthermore, they excreted more 4-pyridoxic acid after vitamin B_6 supplementation than when these women were under the effect of natural ovarian estrogens, indicating that there was a decreased requirement for vitamin B_6 in the presence of the synthetic ethinylestradiol. Under the effect of norethisterone the transaminase enzymes were inhibited, as evidenced by the decreased levels of kynurenic acid and xanthurenic acid. Under the joint effect of ethinylestradiol and norethisterone, the pattern in the preovulatory phase was also corrected. This indicates that the inhibition to the transaminase induced by norethisterone was antagonized and corrected by the synthetic estrogen.

It could be concluded, therefore, that the metabolism of tryptophan is influenced by the physiological variations correlated with the menstrual cycle. Also, the use of this particular oral contraceptive did not lead to accumulation of the carcinogenic tryptophan metabolites.

References

1. KELLER, N., U. I. RICHARDSON AND F. E. YATES. Protein binding and the biological activity of corticosteroids: in vivo induction of hepatic and pancreatic alanine aminotransferase by corticosteroids in normal and estrogen-treated rats. Endocrinology 84: 49, 1969.
2. SINGER, S., AND M. MASON. The effects of the administration of sodium benzoate and diethylstilbestrol disulfate on the hepatic levels of several glucocorticoid-sensitive enzymes in adrenalectomized rats. Biochim. Biophys. Acta 146: 443, 1967.

Effect of an Oral Contraceptive Agent on Blood Pressure Response to Renin

BEN H. DOUGLAS, RICHARD P. HULL, AND HERBERT G. LANGFORD

An occasional patient develops hypertension that appears to be related to the use of oral contraceptive agents (1). There is suggestive evidence linking changes in the renin-angiotensin-aldosterone system to the change in blood pressure. Renin, an enzyme from the kidney, acts on renin substrate, a plasma protein, to release angiotensin, a powerful vasoconstrictor and stimulator of aldosterone secretion. The concentration of renin-substrate is increased by estrogens, and was increased in all patients studied by Laragh with hypertension apparently produced by oral contraceptives (2).

Renin substrate has not been considered to be rate-limiting *in vivo* (3). We have found that rats treated with large amounts of an oral contraceptive had a decreased blood pressure response to angiotensin but an increased blood pressure response to renin, suggesting that renin substrate was rate-limiting *in vivo*.

Materials and Methods. Twenty Holtzman albino female rats, weighing 200 to 250 g, were treated with norethynodrel with mestranol (Enovid R), given orally in their diet, in amounts calculated to give the normal human amount of a weight basis (0.01 mg/kg/day). Twenty additional rats received 10× the normal human amount of Enovid (1.0 mg/kg/day) and 20 untreated rats served as control animals.

After 3 weeks on therapy the rats were anesthetized with 30 mg/kg of sodium pentobarbital and the femoral artery and external jugular vein were cannulated. The blood pressure response to 0.12, 0.25, and 0.50 μg/kg angiotensin (Ciba) was then determined on 10 animals randomly selected from each group.

The blood pressure response to renin was determined on the 10 remaining animals from each group. The renin was prepared by a modification of the method of Haas and Goldblatt (3). Amounts that gave a blood pressure response approximately equal to the 3 dose levels of angiotensin were used. The blood pressure was recorded continuously on a Grass polygraph recorder. The renin and angiotensin were given intravenously.

Results. Figure 1A shows the blood pressure response to angiotensin. The rats which received 1.0 mg/kg/day Enovid (10× dose) had a significant ($p < 0.01$) decrease in their blood pressure response to the largest amount of angiotensin given. There was no significant difference in angiotensin responsiveness between the control group and the animals which received the normal dose (0.1 mg/kg/day) of Enovid.

Figure 1B shows the blood pressure response to renin. A completely different pattern of response is now evident. There was a significant ($p < 0.01$) increase in blood pressure response to all doses of renin in the rats treated with 1.0 mg/kg/day Enovid (10× normal dose). The animals which received the normal dose of Enovid appeared to have a decreased blood pressure response to renin but the differences were not significant.

Discussion. The changes produced by estrogens and progestational agents are complex and may have opposing influences on vascular and electrolyte homeostasis. Estrogen may cause sodium retention directly by action on the kidney, and indirectly by increasing venous volume (4, 5). Progestational agents are said to cause sodium excretion (6). Estrogens increase renin-substrate (3), and the progestogen, norethynodrel, increases aldosterone secretion (7). This study demonstrates that angiotensin responsiveness is decreased, as it is in many conditions where renin is increased.

The complexity of the changes produced by oral contraceptives makes it difficult to state the precise cause of the hypertension occasionally found in association with their use. Two conclusions can be drawn from the studies reported here. First, renin substrate is apparently rate-limiting *in vivo* in the blood pressure response to exogenous renin, thus confirming the suggestion of Laragh (2). Secondly, measurement of renin levels may not give a true guide to angiotensin production. Also, as angiotensin responsiveness can be reduced by oral contraceptive agents, determination of both angiotensin levels and angiotensin responsiveness is necessary before the role of changes in the renin-angiotensin system in the genesis of oral contraceptive-produced hypertension can be evaluated.

It is probable that the changes in renin responsiveness found in this study would be present with any oral contraceptive containing estrogens and progestins. Similar studies with agents containing only progestins are planned.

Summary. Rats were treated with norethyn-

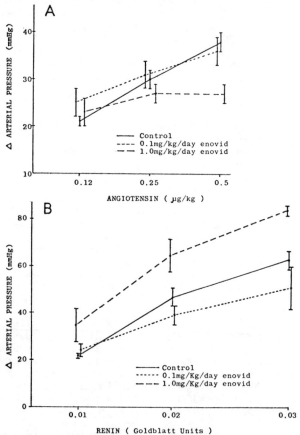

FIG. 1. The effect of chronic Enovid administration on the blood pressure response to angiotensin (A), and renin (B) is shown. Standard errors of the mean are indicated.

odrel with mestranol given orally mixed with their diet in amounts calculated to give 1 and 10✕ the normal human amount on a weight basis. The animals which received 10✕ normal norethynodrel–mestranol had a significant decrease in their blood pressure response to the largest amount of angiotensin and a significant increase in their blood pressure response to renin. These data indicate that renin substrate is rate-limiting *in vivo*.

We acknowledge the technical assistance of Mrs. Jo Ann Douglas and the helpful advice of Dr. Victor Drill of the G. D. Searle Company.

1. Newton, M., Sealey, J., and Ledingham, J., Amer. J. Obstet. Gynecol. 101, 1037 (1968).

2. Laragh, J., Sealey, J., Ledingham, J., and Newton, M., J. Amer. Med. Ass. 201, 918 (1967).

3. Haas, E., and Goldblatt, H., Circ. Res. 20, 45 (1967).

4. Dignam, W. S., Voskian, J., and Assali, N. S., J. Clin. Endocrinol. 16, Metab. 1032 (1956).

5. Ueland, K., and Parer, J., Amer. J. Obstet. Gynecol. 96, 400 (1966).

6. Katz, F., and Kappas, A., J. Clin. Invest. 46, 1768 (1967).

7. Laidlaw, J. C., Ruse, J. L., and Gornall, A. G., J. Clin. Endocrinol. Metab. 22, 161 (1962).

The Effect of Enovid on the Binding of Thyroxine To Plasma Proteins *In Vitro*

HENRY A. MOSES, PH.D., CLINTON BATTLE AND DOTTIE WATSON

POPULATION control by means of limiting the number of births is an obviously desirable mechanism in combating over-population. More than a dozen antifertility steroids in combination or sequential dosages have been placed on the drug market since *Enovid* (G. D. Searle preparation of norethynodrel, and mestranol) was introduced in 1960.

The mechanism of action of these drugs remains relatively obscure and an array of pharmacologic effects have been observed in clinical studies and in laboratory investigations.

The use of oral contraceptives (antifertility preparations) is safe according to a report released in the summer of 1969, but there is a growing concern over the side effects of "The Pill."[1] British investigators have for three years found repeatedly that there is an increase in some thromboembolic disorders in women taking the medications.[2, 3, 4]

Long-term administration of oral contraceptives has been shown to interfere with various aspects of hepatic function in women. Among the parameters which were measured showing alterations were a decrease execretory capacity of bromosulfonphthalein.

Using the white rat as the experimental animal and the *Enovid* preparation, it has been found that ovulation is inhibited by the drug and this inhibition of ovulation is associated with the development of follicular cysts within the ovary. The size of the liver was increased in animals given the drug. One of the striking observations in the experimental animals was the increase noted in the size of the thyroid gland. It has been known for many years that there exists more than a casual relationship between the sex hormones and the thyroid hormones. During pregnancy, the thyroid gland becomes enlarged and the protein bound iodine (PBI) level is elevated—often to twice its normal value. The basal body temperature is closely associated with ovulation. Ovulation day is determined as the day with the lowest basal temperature immediately preceding several days of sustained elevation of basal temperature which is followed by a menstrual flow.

The administration of thyroxine to rats which had been given a dosage of *Enovid* previously shown to be adequate to cause ovarian cysts, prevented the formation of these cysts. Polycystic ovaries may be induced in the rat by giving human chorionic gonadotrophin (HCG) after inducing a state of hypothyroidism using thiouracil.

Investigations in this laboratory have been concerned with two aspects of antifertility drug use: 1) the thromboembolic phenomenon associated with the oral contraceptives and 2) the effect of these steroids on thyroxine metabolism.

The purpose of this investigation was to determine if *Enovid* altered the binding of thyroxine to plasma proteins in vitro.

MATERIAL AND METHODS

A column containing Sephadex G-25-40 which had been made into a slurry using a 0.15M, pH 7.4 trihydroxymethylamino methane (tris) buffer was constructed. The column measured 15.0 centimeters in height and had a diameter of 1.3 centimeters. Tris was chosen over other buffer systems due to the fact that residual binding of thyroxine by the Sephadex particles is least using this buffer system as compared to phosphate, according to Levin and Linde.[5]

A 0.2 ml. aliquot of diagnostic plasma was placed on the column and eluted with tris buffer. Aliquots of one milliliter volume were collected and the protein present measured using the Lowry procedure.[6] I^{131} thyroxine (Abbott Laboratories) with 0.55 mc activity in a volume of 1.83 mls. (50% propyleneglycol) was diluted to 2.0 mls. using tris buffer, 0.15M, pH 7.4.

Samples of diagnostic plasma (Warner-Chilcott) were reconstituted (solubilized) and a constant amount of I^{131} labeled thyroxine which was adequate to give a statistically sufficient amount of ionizing radiation as detected on the counting system available was added to the solubilized plasma. Varying amounts of *Enovid* which had been solubilized in 0.1M phosphate buffer pH 7.4 in 5% ethanol, as indicated in Table 1 were added to the reconstituted plasma, keeping the volumes constant by using the tris buffer.

Each vial of plasma with the thyroxine and *Enovid* were allowed to equilibrate at room temperature for 60 minutes after which 0.2 mls were placed on the column and eluted with tris buffer. Another 0.2 ml aliquot was placed on a planchet, evaporated to dryness on a hot plate and counted as a reference standard. This enabled the calculation of the per cent of the applied sample which was protein bound and free and avoided the necessity of calculating and making corrections for radioactive decay. The eluant was collected in one milliliter fractions and of this volume, 0.2 ml from each tube was placed on a planchet and evaporated to dryness. The protein was determined in a one-half milliliter volume of each aliquot collected from the column. Between each run on the column, a 5 ml. aliquot of a 2% human albumin solution was used to flush the column of any residual isotope that may have remained.

The radioactivity associated with the fractions of eluant which contained protein and the radioactivity found in the non-protein containing fractions were compared and the ratios calculated for each run. The total amount of radioactivity recovered of the 0.2 ml. aliquot placed on the column was determined.

RESULTS AND DISCUSSION

Of the total amount of I^{131} added to the column more than 90% could be recovered by the time the volume of eluant representing the internal volume had flowed through the column. This good recovery was not altered by the presence of *Enovid*, nevertheless, the columns were always flushed with 5 mls. of the two per cent albumin and re-equilibrated with the tris buffer before a subsequent run was made.

Based on the radioactivity associated with the protein and that which came off the column as

TABLE 1.—COMPOSITION OF TEST SOLUTIONS BINDING OF THYROXINE

Run No.	Enovid (μgm)	$I^{131}μc$	Diag-nostic Plasma – mls	Tris Buffer to a Total Volume – mls
A	0	0.5	0.5	2.0
B	50	0.5	0.5	2.0
C	100	0.5	0.5	2.0
D	200	0.5	0.5	2.0

I^{131} labeled free thyroxine, it appears that the drug preparation markedly increased the binding of the thyroxine to the plasma protein. The results are presented in Table 2. Some researchers have concluded that the major factor associated with the increased PBI observed during pregnancy and in the use of oral contraceptives is the increase in plasma protein, especially albumin.[7] It is possible that aside from the increased protein content the estrogen-progestogen preparation has a direct effect on the binding *in vivo* as is observed *in vitro*. Also, one plausible explanation as to the increased thyroid size in animals receiving the *Enovid* preparation may be due to the fact that less thyroxine is physiologically active (in the free form) in the presence of *Enovid* in the plasma, hence, the gland secretes more thyroxine as manifested by its increased size.[8, 9]

TABLE 2.—EFFECT OF ENOVID ON BINDING OF THYROXINE - I^{131} TO PLASMA PROTEINS

Run No.	Enovid (μgm)	% Isotope Recovered	Ratio Bound $T_4 I^{131}$ / Free $T_4 I^{131}$
A	0	94	1.7
B	50	93	2.5
C	100	95	3.2
D	200	93	6.0

CONCLUSIONS

Sephadex G-25-40 was successfully used to separate protein bound thyroxine from free thyroxine and the distribution of the two forms of thyroxine was followed using the radioisotopic tracer thyroxine labeled I^{131}.

Enovid (norethynodrel-mestranol) increased the extent to which human plasma proteins bound thyroxine.

LITERATURE CITED

1. The Pill: FDA Calls It Safe. Chem. and Engin. News, 47:16, 1969.
2. Investigation of Relationship between Use of Oral Contraceptives and Thromboembolic Diseases VESSEY, M. and R. DOLL. Brit. Med. J., 2:199-205, 1968.
3. Oral Contraceptives and Thromboembolic Disease DRILL, V. and D. CALHOUN. J. A. M. A., 206:77-84, 1968.
4. Effects of Low Dose Oral Contraceptives on Blood Coagulation POLLER, L., A. TABIOWO, and J. THOMSON. Brit. Med. J., 3:218-219, 1968.
5. Binding of Thyroxine to Human Serum Proteins LEVIN, K. and S. LINDE. Scand. J. Clin. and Lab. Invest., 69:76, 1963.
6. Protein Measurement with the Folin Phenol Reagent LOWRY, O. H., and N. J. ROSEBROUGH, A. L. FARR, and R. J. RANDALL. J. Biol. Chem. 183:265, 1951.
7. WILLIAMS, R. H. Textbook of Endocrinology. W. B. Saunders Co., Phila., 1962, p. 130.
8. Further Studies of An Antifertility Preparation MOSES, H. A. and H. M. FRAZIER. J. N. M. A., 59:332, 1967.
9. MOSES, H. A., and J. K. WINFIELD, H. M. FRAZIER, and J. C. ASHHURST. Thyroxine Antifertility Steroid Interrelations in the Albino Rat. J. N. M. A., 61:13, 1969.

Carbohydrate Metabolism in Long-Term Oral Contraceptive Users

ABELARDO FUERTES-DE LA HABA, MD, DPH, FACOG,
GLORIA VEGA-DE RODRIGUEZ, MD and
IVÁN PELEGRINA, MD, MPH, FACOG

S EVERAL MILLION WOMEN all over the world are using oral estrogen-progestin medication for contraceptive purposes. During the years 1956–1962, a group of Puerto Rican women were first given these progestational agents for contraception continuously for periods ranging up to 13 years.[1-3]

Studies on alterations in carbohydrate metabolism after short- and long-term use of these drugs are numerous.[4-7] In general, they suggest that carbohydrate tolerance is impaired and that the oral glucose tolerance test appears to be altered more than is the intravenous. Furthermore, insulin and growth hormone levels have been found to be elevated.[8-9] Posner et al have reported that the effect of the drug on the intravenous glucose tolerance test tapers after the first six months of therapy.[10] The significance of these abnormalities and their effects in the patient developing overt diabetes, with or without its complications, is yet to be elucidated. If the improvement in carbohydrate tolerance is due to chronic pancreatic stimulation, as suggested by elevated insulin values, exhaustion of the pancreas with the development of overt diabetes should be expected.

For this reason, we decided to study carbohydrate tolerance in a group of patients who have been taking a combination of estrogen-progestin ever since they were first made available to our group for study.

MATERIALS AND METHODS

STUDY GROUP. During the years 1956–1962 a total of 836 patients were admitted to our clinic in Rio Piedras, Puerto Rico for field trials with Enovid.* This is the original

Appreciation is expressed to Dr. Ishver Bangdiwala, Professor of Statistics, Graduate School, University of Puerto Rico, and Dr. J. J. Hernandez-Cibes, Associate Professor in Obstetrics and Gynecology, for their helpful advice and cooperation.

Supported by Grant 680-0710A from the Ford Foundation.

Appreciation is expressed to G. D. Searle and Co. for supplying Enovid.

---

* Norethynodrel-mestranol-Searle.

27

group of García, Pincus and Rock, and has since been called Old Enovid. Fifty-three of these patients are still taking some form of Enovid and constitute our study group. A comparison of the main characteristics of the whole group (836) and of the study group (53) was made. No statistical difference was found when the following characteristics were compared: age, weight, height, parity and education. These women have been taking contraceptive medication for a total of 8111 cycles, average 122 cycles, arithmetic mean 120.8 cycles, range 62–183, estimated standard deviation 33.4 cycles, and standard error of the mean 4.6 (Table 1). The average dose of steroid has been 3.72 mg per day, per cycle (±0.18 SE). The dosage distribution is given in Table 2.

TABLE 1. NUMBER OF CONTRACEPTIVE MEDICATION CYCLES TAKEN BY OLD ENOVID GROUP

Total No. of patients	*Enovid 10 mg	Enovid 5 mg	Enovid-E 2.5 mg	Total No. of cycles
19	349	1837	716	2902
20	0	1056	2709	3765
14	0	0	1444	1444
53	349	2893	4869	8111

* Norethynodrel, 9.85 mg; mestranol, .15mg; total steroid, 10 mg/tablet Norethynodrel, 5 mg; mestranol, .075 mg; total steroid 5.075 mg/tablet Norethynodrel, 2.5 mg; mestranol, 0.1 mg; total steroid 2.6 mg/tablet

TABLE 2. AVERAGE DOSE PER DAY PER CYCLE TAKEN BY PATIENTS IN THE STUDY GROUP

Dose (mg)	2.1–3.0	3.1–4.0	4.1–5.0	5.1–6.0	6.1–7.0
No. of patients	28	2	14	7	2

(Statistical method used was the Student *t* test).

After a complete history had been taken, each patient was given a physical examination by an endocrinologist in association with the gynecologist. Particular care was taken in obtaining an accurate history of diabetes: family history, infant birth weights, toxemia, unexplained stillbirths, neonatal deaths, and in observing physical findings that could be related to diabetes. No patient gave a history of diabetes and all 53 patients were submitted to an oral glucose tolerance test.

The oral glucose tolerance test was done according to procedure recommended.[12] All subjects were given a 3-day, 300g carbohydrate preparatory diet. The test was done after a glucose overload of 30 g/sq m of body surface was given in the form of a carbonated drink.* Fasting, 1- 2- and 3-hour samples were drawn. Blood was drawn from the antecubital vein into fluoride tubes, and the glucose content analyzed in a Technicon. Autoanalyzer using a glucose oxidase method. The test was performed at any time after the patient had taken at least 5 Enovid tablets but before she stopped them for that cycle (tablet days 5–18). This was done to assure that she was taking medication and to prevent any variation that may occur on the days she is not taking tablets.

The results were interpreted as follows: any subject in whom the sum of the four glucose values was above 500 mg was considered abnormal. Any patient with values between 425–499 was retested with cortisone.[13] This test was done at least 3 days after the last tablet of one cycle and before the first tablet of the next cycle in order to eliminate, as much as possible the potentiating effect of estrogen-progestin medication on the cortisone glucose tolerance test.

RESULTS

Thirty of the 53 patients were classified as normal and 23 as prediabetic on the basis of their histories (Table 3). Six patients were found to have blood pressures of 140/90 mm Hg or over and their hypertensive status is being studied. There were no patients with evidence of neuropathy or

* Glucola,® Ames Company, Elkhart, Indiana.

TABLE 3. CLASSIFICATION OF STUDY GROUP

1—Normal	30
2—Prediabetic	23
Family history	Positive
Father	4
Mother	6
Both parents	4
Other	2
Obstetric history	
Large babies	12
Stillborn or neonatal deaths	5

diabetic retinopathy and no patient gave a history of renal disease.

GENERAL. Twelve of the 53 patients (22.6%) had an abnormal carbohydrate tolerance. Of these 12, two (3.77%) were classified as overt diabetics, five (9.43%) had an abnormal glucose tolerance test and 5 others had an abnormal cortisone tolerance test.

NORMAL GROUP. Four (13.3%) of the 30 patients who had been considered normal had an abnormal carbohydrate tolerance. Of these 4, one (3.3%) had an abnormal glucose tolerance test and three (10%) had an abnormal cortisone tolerance test (Table 4).

PREDIABETIC GROUP. Eight of the 23 patients (34.8%) in the prediabetic group were considered to have an abnormal carbohydrate tolerance. Of these 8, two (8.7%) were considered overt diabetics; 4 (17.4%) had abnormal GTT and 2 (8.7%) had an abnormal cortisone tolerance test (Table 5).

DIABETIC GROUP. Two of the patients were considered to be overt diabetics. These 2 patients denied being diabetics in their initial histories and had been included in the prediabetic group (see above). Both did not mention their diabetes because they would be denied the contraceptive medication. The glucose tolerance tests are summarized in Table 6. The history of these 2 patients is very significant, however, and is, therefore, summarized here:

CFC was a 34-year-old, gravida 4, para 3, abortion 1 (ectopic), neonatal death 1, stillborn 1 (12 lb), whose father, grandfather, and aunt are known diabetics. She was diagnosed as having gestational diabetes in 1957; gave birth to her only living child, an 8-pound baby at 36 wks gestation by cesarean section. She required 60 U NPH during the pregnancy. She was told

TABLE 4. ABNORMAL GLUCOSE TOLERANCE AND CORTISONE GLUCOSE TOLERANCE IN NORMAL GROUP

				Glucose tolerance								
				Oral					Cortisone			
Patient No.	Age	Height	Weight	F	1	2	3	S	F	1	2	3
493	44	55	161	98	136	173	122	529				
283	41	61	115	86	161	123	72	438	168	286	275	191
426	37	60	146	93	166	101	97	457	120	230	170	142
143	33	60	143	86	159	122	73	440	113	210	151	128

TABLE 5. ABNORMAL GLUCOSE TOLERANCE AND CORTISONE GLUCOSE TOLERANCE IN THE PREDIABETIC GROUP

				Glucose tolerance tests								
				Oral					Cortisone			
Patient No.	Age	Height	Weight	F	1hr	2hrs	3hrs	S	F	1hr	2hrs	3hrs
325	46	59	140	110	194	171	103	578				
509	38	58	138	100	125	138	152	515				
645	27	60	135	106	172	130	109	517				
685	33	59	153	121	276	155	094	646				
694	43	63	146	096	166	132	075	469	122	183	190	139
826	29	58	116	090	151	119	066	426	114	212	194	123

Patient No.	Age	Height	Weight	Oral					Cortisone			
				F	1	2	3	S	F	1	2	3
427	35	63	137	292	358	380	334	1364				
396	34	62	134	76	158	158	100	491	102	202	201	227

to maintain a blood sugar of 200 mg/100 ml postpartum and insulin was prescribed for her but she did not use it and did not follow any dietary regime. She was given contraceptive therapy in 1958. This history was withheld, at that time. She now has completed 149 cycles on Enovid. Physical examination and laboratory tests show no evidence of retinopathy, neuropathy, vascular disease or nephropathy. Fasting blood sugar values were around 200 mg/100 ml during the study period.

ICH, age 33, gravida 2, para 2, one baby 9½ lb. Her father, mother, maternal grandmother and two siblings are diabetics. She has been taking Enovid for 152 cycles (almost 13 years). She was first told that she had diabetes 3 years ago after the death of her mother, and has been on a diet since then, maintaining a normal fasting blood sugar: her original glucose tolerance test was doubtful, sum 491. The cortisone test was abnormal. She had no evidence of retinopathy, neuropathy, vascular disease or nephropathy.

As may be seen from the case summaries, one of the patients was already a diabetic when she began the tablets. Her diabetes has been rather stable with a blood sugar around 200 mg/100 ml, and there is no clinical evidence of diabetic complications. She refuses to stop taking the contraceptives and does not desire sterilization. Improvement of diabetes with estrogen therapy has been reported previously.[14] This patient has not shown improvement but neither has her diabetes progressed, in spite of the fact that she does not follow any diabetic regime.

The other patient had a very strong family history of diabetes; one brother is a diabetic at age 39, a sister at age 42. Her diagnosis was made after the death of her mother and she now maintains a normal fasting blood

sugar on diet only. This history is rather typical of many diabetics.

DISCUSSION

There is no doubt that oral contraceptive medication is a highly effective method of fertility control. Reports on the metabolic abnormalities elicited by its use suggest that the progestational steroids may be diabetogenic. Most of the data presented show a rather early and persistent alteration of the oral glucose tolerance in women taking oral contraceptives. The effect of continuous and prolonged use of these drugs could be construed as producing clinical diabetes mellitus with its complications.

Our study group of 53 patients has been taking high-dosage medication for continuous prolonged periods. The least number of consecutive cycles taken by our patients is equivalent to 5 years, while some of them have been using continuous contraception for over 13 years. This study was particularly intended to determine whether such prolonged and continuous use of high-dosage medication would, in effect, be a causative factor in the development of overt diabetes mellitus with or without complications.

Two of the 53 patients (3.77%) were found to have clinical diabetes mellitus. One of the 2 patients was a diabetic before she began to receive contraceptive therapy. Her diabetes has not deteriorated and she has not developed complications, in spite of continuous medication. The remaining patient (1.9%) gives a rather classical history of diabetes. At present, she maintains a normal

30

glucose tolerance on diet only. Her opportunities for developing diabetes, in view of her family history, would have been almost 100% whether she had taken contraceptive tablets or not.

In these 2 patients, contraceptive medication can not be related in cause-and-effect terms to the diabetic state nor to its aggravation, since 1 patient was already a diabetic and the other had a family history highly compatible with the development of this disease. In neither of these two patients has the medication aggravated their diabetic condition.

Five other patients (9.43%) had an abnormal glucose tolerance. This figure is lower than that usually reported for abnormal tolerance with the use of progestational agents. Four of these patients had been classified as prediabetics. They represent 19% of the prediabetic group. All had at least one diabetic parent. The genetic susceptibility to diabetes when one parent is a diabetic is around 22%.[15] One patient with an abnormal tolerance had been classified in the normal group. She is obese and an abnormal tolerance has been reported in obese individuals.

The cortisone glucose tolerance test proved to be abnormal in all patients upon whom it was done. The test in still considered a research tool and its evaluation may be misleading in patients taking oral contraceptives. Our aim is to follow these patients to determine if they will eventually develop diabetes or if this is a result of the combination of progestational agent with cortisone.

In summary, we can state that only one patient (1.9%) in the total group has developed clinical diabetes. She has shown no complications. One additional patient, who was already a diabetic, has not developed complications nor has her diabetes progressed. Five additional patients (9.4%) maintain an abnormal glucose tolerance but have not developed any evidence of overt diabetes or its complications. The 7 patients represent 13.2% of the total group.

REFERENCES

1. Pincus G, Rock J, Garcia CR: Effects of certain 19- nor steroids upon reproductive processes. Ann NY Acad Sci 71:677–690, 1958
2. Rice-Wray E: Field study with Enovid as a contraceptive agent, 19-nor Progestational Steroids. Chicago, GD Searle, 1957, p 78–85
3. García CR, Pincus G, Rock J: Effects of three 19-nor steroids on human ovulation and menstruation. Amer J Obstet Gynec 75:82–97, 1958
4. Gershberg H, Javier Z, Hulse M: Glucose tolerance in women receiving an ovulatory suppressant. Diabetes 13:4, 378–382, 1964
5. Wynn V, Doar JWH: Some effects of oral contraceptives on carbohydrate metabolism. Lancet 2:715–719, 1966
6. Posner NA, Silverstone FA, Pomerance W, Baumgold D: Oral contraceptives and intravenous glucose tolerance. I. Data noted early in treatment. Obstet Gynec 29: 79–86, 1967
7. Javier Z, Gershberg H, Hulse M: Ovulatory suppressants, estrogen, and carbohydrate metabolism. Metabolism 17:443–456, 1968
8. Spellacy WN, Carlson KL: Plasma insulin and blood glucose levels in patients taking oral contraceptives. Amer J Obstet Gynec 95:474–478, 1966
9. Yen SSC, Vela P: Carbohydrate metabolism and long-term use of contraceptives. J Repro Med 3:6–18, 1969
10. Posner NA, Silverstone FA, Singer N: Intravenous glucose tolerance: II. Long term effect. Obstet Gynec 29:187–92, 1967
11. Drill VA: Endocrine properties and long-term safety of oral contraceptives Metabolism 14: 295, 1965
12. Standardization of the GTT—Report of Committee on Statistics. Diabetes 18:299–307, 1969
13. Fajans S, Conn JW: An Approach to the prediction of diabetes mellitus by modification of the glucose tolerance test with cortisone. Diabetes 3:296–304, 1954
14. Gershberg H, Javier Z, Hulse M, et al: Improvement of glucose tolerance with estrogen treatment in maturity on set diabetes. Program of the Twenty-seventh Meeting of the American Diabetes Association, June 1967
15. Stunberg AG: Heredity in diabetes mellitus. Diabetes 10:269–74, 1961
16. Diabetes Source Book, US Department of Health Education and Welfare, Public Health Service. Publication No 1168, May 1964

REDUCTION OF PLASMA TYROSINE BY ORAL CONTRACEPTIVES AND OESTROGENS: A POSSIBLE CONSEQUENCE OF TYROSINE AMINOTRANSFERASE INDUCTION

D. P. ROSE and D. G. CRAMP

The use of combined oestrogen–progestogen preparations for contraceptive purposes is accompanied by a wide range of metabolic changes, most of which appear to be due to the oestrogen component.[1] The administration of oestrogens causes a rise in the level of plasma cortisol, and Wynn and Doar[2,3] have suggested that both the impairment of glucose tolerance and the raised blood pyruvate levels which occur in women taking the combined type of oral contraceptives are a consequence of increased adrenal glucocorticoid activity.

The level of tyrosine aminotransferase in rat liver is increased by adrenocorticosteroids, and in man the reduced level of tyrosine in plasma following treatment with cortisone has also been attributed to elevated activity of this enzyme[4]. If the level of physiologically active cortisol is raised in women taking contraceptive steroids, they too may have elevated liver tyrosine aminotransferase activity. Therefore, we have determined the plasma tyrosine in a group of women before and after the administration of an oestrogen–progestogen preparation, and in 2 women treated with oestrogen alone.

SUBJECTS AND METHODS

Fasting plasma tyrosine levels were determined for 23 women before they start-

32

ed to use an oral contraceptive and again when they had been taking such a steroid preparation for at least 3 months. Six different contraceptives, all of the combined oestrogen–progestogen type, were included in the study. The effect of an oestrogen alone was observed in 2 female volunteers. In one case ethinyl oestradiol was given orally in a dose of o.1 mg daily for 22 days. Plasma tyrosine levels were determined before starting oestrogen administration, at intervals throughout treatment, and then until the effect of the hormone was no longer apparent. For the second study the plasma tyrosine was determined in two samples obtained before treatment and again after 7 and 14 days of ethinyl oestradiol administration in a daily dose of o.1 mg.

Plasma tyrosine was determined by the fluorimetric method of Waalkes and Udenfriend[5], using samples of heparinized blood obtained after an overnight fast.

RESULTS

The plasma tyrosine levels of the 23 women before taking an oral contraceptive ranged from 8.1–31.1 μg/ml (mean 13.0 $\pm$ SD 5.4). Except for an extremely obese woman with a level of 31.1 μg/ml, these control values agreed well with the normal range obtained by Rivlin and Melmon[4]. When taking an oral contraceptive, the plasma tyrosine ranged from 7.1–15.3 μg/ml (mean 9.0 $\pm$ SD 2.3). The overall difference between the control values and those during oral contraceptive administration was highly significant ($P < 0.001$). 20 of the 23 women showed a reduction of the plasma tyrosine level when they were taking an oral contraceptive; in 3 there was no change (Fig. 1). The changes were not associated with the use of any particular oestrogen–progestogen combination, nor were they related to an alteration in body weight during the period of administration.

In the first study with an oestrogen alone the plasma tyrosine showed a marked reduction 48 h after commencing treatment with ethinyl oestradiol, and there was an

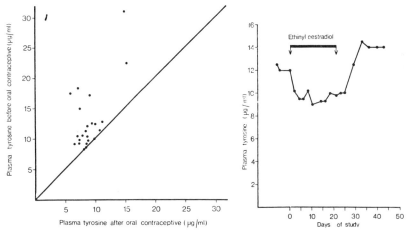

Fig. 1. The plasma tyrosine levels of 23 women before and after the administration of a combined oestrogen–progestogen oral contraceptive. Points above the 45° line indicate a reduction in plasma tyrosine after taking an oral contraceptive.

Fig. 2. The effect of ethinyl oestradiol, o.1 mg daily, on the plasma tyrosine level.

33

equally prompt return to the pretreatment level at the end of the period of hormone administration. This was followed by a further rise to levels in excess of those observed before giving the steroid (Fig. 2). The second subject who was treated with ethinyl oestradiol also showed a reduction of plasma tyrosine; the pretreatment values were 12.5 and 12.2 μg/ml, after 7 days of oestrogen the level was 10.0 μg/ml, and after 14 days it was 9.1 μg/ml.

DISCUSSION

Craft and Wise[6,7] have found that the total plasma amino acid level, as measured by the determination of α-amino nitrogen, is reduced in women taking oestrogen–progestogen preparations, and also immediately following ovulation in those who are not using oral contraceptives. They suggest that these changes are due to an anabolic effect of the progestogenic component. Zinneman et al.[8] have studied the effect of progesterone, given alone or in combination with stilboestrol, upon both the individual plasma and urinary free amino acids, determined by automatic amino acid analysis. The daily administration of 100 mg progesterone for 7 days produced a significant decrease in the plasma concentrations of threonine, alanine, cystine, ornithine and arginine, and an increase of phenylalanine. The only urinary changes were increases of taurine and phenylalanine. When 4 months later a combination of 100 mg progesterone and 5 mg stilboestrol was given daily for 7 days, there were significant decreases in the plasma levels of serine, citrulline, glycine, alanine, valine, ornithine, lysine and arginine, but significant increases only in urinary taurine, valine and cystathionine. The mean value for the tyrosine concentration in plasma was reduced and in urine it was increased, but the changes were not statistically significant. These observations of reduced plasma amino acid levels without corresponding urinary losses are consistent with an anabolic effect of progesterone and a resulting increased amino acid utilization by the liver.

Zinneman et al.[9], however, have also examined the effect of stilboestrol alone on amino acid levels. When 5 mg was given daily for 5 days there were significant decreases of plasma tyrosine, glutamic acid and ornithine. There were increases in urinary glutamic acid and ornithine, and although these did not reach levels of statistical significance this suggests that the reduced plasma levels of these amino acids were due to a renal loss. However, the urinary excretion of tyrosine was significantly decreased, and as Zinneman and coworkers pointed out, this, combined with the low plasma tyrosine, implies a prerenal effect of oestrogens on tyrosine metabolism.

Thus, although the principal factor responsible for the reduced *total* plasma amino acid level in women taking oral contraceptives may be the progestogenic component, as proposed by Craft and Wise[7], it does appear that the oestrogen produces a fall in the plasma levels of specific amino acids. The present work has shown that this is true of tyrosine, and oral contraceptives and oestrogens alone have been shown also to enhance the hepatic metabolism of tryptophan along the degradative pathway leading to nicotinic acid ribonucleotide synthesis[10–12].

The administration of oestrogens produces an elevated level of plasma 17-hydroxycorticosteroids[13], and a similar change occurs in women who are taking oestrogen–progestogen preparations for contraceptive purposes. Although most of this increased circulating steroid is protein-bound, and in the past has been considered

34

generally to be physiologically inert, there is also a small rise in the unbound, free plasma cortisol[14]. Further, recent work by Keller et al.[15] has shown a rise in plasma 17-hydroxycorticosteroids due to oestrogen administration will cause an elevation in the activity of the cortisol-inducible enzyme alanine aminotransferase in rat liver. They suggest that the protein-bound steroid is able to pass through the plasma membrane of the hepatic cell, by pinocytosis, and there dissociate from the binding globulin to yield the active corticosteroid. If such a mechanism is responsible for the elevated level of hepatic alanine aminotransferase then similar changes may be expected in the activity of other liver enzymes that are known to be inducible by adrenal corticosteroids. This possibility has been discussed previously with regard to tryptophan oxygenase and the abnormal tryptophan metabolism which occurs in women taking oral contraceptives[16].

Tyrosine aminotransferase catalyzes the initial step in tyrosine degradation and its activity is markedly elevated by corticosteroids[17]. Glucocorticoids also reduce the level of plasma tyrosine in both the rat and man, and this effect has been ascribed to an increased rate of degradation of the amino acid by tyrosine aminotransferase[18,4]. A renal loss of tyrosine is not responsible for the low plasma level because although large doses of cortisol do produce an aminoaciduria the urinary excretion of tyrosine remains within normal limits[19].

We conclude from the present study that the plasma tyrosine levels of women taking oral contraceptives are reduced, that this effect is due to the oestrogenic component, and that the likely mechanism is an increased activity in hepatic tyrosine aminotransferase induced by elevated levels of cortisol.

We have no explanation for the rise in plasma tyrosine to a level in excess of the pretreatment value when the ethinyl estradiol was discontinued (Fig. 2), but it is of interest that a similar effect was obtained 24 h after a 5-day period of cortisol administration[19].

ACKNOWLEDGEMENT

We thank Professor Victor Wynn for his help and interest in this study.
The work was supported through Contract No. Ph-43-67-1344 of the U.S. National Institutes of Health.

REFERENCES

1 H. A. SALHANICK, D. M. KIPNIS AND R. L. VANDE WIELE (Eds.), Metabolic Effects of Gonadal Hormones and Contraceptive Steroids, Plenum Publishing Co., New York, 1969.
2 V. WYNN AND J. W. H. DOAR, Lancet, ii (1966) 715.
3 V. WYNN AND J. W. H. DOAR, Lancet, ii (1969) 761.
4 R. S. RIVLIN AND K. L. MELMON, J. Clin. Invest., 44 (1965) 1960.
5 T. P. WAALKES AND S. J. UDENFRIEND, J. Lab. Clin. Med., 50 (1957) 733.
6 I. L. CRAFT AND I. WISE, Nature, 222 (1969) 487.
7 I. L. CRAFT AND I. WISE, Lancet, ii (1969) 1138.
8 H. H. ZINNEMAN, U. S. SEAL AND R. P. DOE, J. Clin. Endocrinol. Metab., 27 (1967) 397.
9 H. H. ZINNEMAN, B. U. MUSA AND R. P. DOE, Metabolism, 14 (1965) 1214.
10 D. P. ROSE, Clin. Sci., 31 (1966) 265.
11 D. P. ROSE, Clin. Chim. Acta, 18 (1967) 221.
12 D. P. ROSE, R. R. BROWN AND J. M. PRICE, Nature, 219 (1968) 1259.
13 A. A. SANDBERG AND W. R. SLAUNWHITE Jr., J. Clin. Invest., 38 (1959) 1290.
14 C. W. BURKE, Brit. Med. J., i (1969) 798.

15 N. KELLER, U. I. RICHARDSON AND F. E. YATES, *Endocrinology*, 84 (1969) 49.
16 D. P. ROSE, *Lancet*, ii (1969) 321.
17 E. C. C. LIN AND W. E. KNOX, *Biochim. Biophys. Acta*, 26 (1957) 85.
18 J. J. BETHEIL, M. FEIGELSON AND P. FEIGELSON, *Biochim. Biophys. Acta*, 105 (1965) 92.
19 H. H. ZINNEMAN, J. J. JOHNSON AND U. S. SEAL, *J. Clin. Endocrinol. Metab.*, 23 (1963) 996.

Estrogen therapy and glucose tolerance test

G. di PAOLA, M.D.

M. ROBIN, M.D.

R. NICHOLSON, M.D.

SINCE THE BEGINNING of oral contraceptive therapy, numerous papers have been published, some outlining its efficiency, others pointing out the undesirable side effects, such as digestive disturbances, weight increase, headaches, or menstrual alterations. Even so, until 1964, little was known of the pharmacologic effects of estrogen-progestin therapy on carbohydrate metabolism, although its action in a way imitates pregnancy, which in itself implies a diabetic tendency. At that time, Gerschberg, Javier, and Hulse[3] found reduced tolerance to glucose in young women taking contraceptive pills containing 5 mg. norethynodrel and 75 γ mestranol, a feature that became more evident in women with family histories of diabetes. The tests were performed in a sufficiently large number of patients—59—but unfortunately these women had not undergone previous tests.

This investigation was supported by a grant from Eli Lilly & Company.

Later Wynn and Doar[21] confirmed the results of Gerschberg, Javier, and Hulse in 105 patients with contraceptive therapy. Abnormal levels were found in 18 per cent and 15 per cent of oral and intravenous tests, respectively. When Buchler and Warren[1] administered stilbestrol or mestranol combined with norethynodrel to 14 menopausal women results of oral glucose tolerance tests were abnormal in 11 instances whereas those of intravenous tests were all within normal values. Spellacy and Carlson,[18] studying 25 young women with a therapeutic regimen of 10 mg. norethynodrel combined with 150 γ mestranol for 20 days found alterations in both the glucose tolerance test and in insulin blood content and attributed these results to pancreatic hyperfunction.

Spellacy, Carlson, and Birk[19] with the same therapeutic regimen in a prolonged treatment of up to 6 weeks found normal blood glucose levels but persistence of elevated insulin values.

Posner and associates,[14] in a recent study of 40 young women, encountered reduced tolerance to intravenous glucose administration during the first 6 months of treatment with Enovid, but this abnormality tended to disappear in 10 patients during an 18 month follow-up. Women using intrauterine contraceptive devices (IUCD) only, and not receiving estrogen therapy, were studied as controls; they had absolutely no alterations in glucose tolerance.

The authors we mentioned above employed a combination of estrogen and progestin; the altered laboratory findings, however, have been mainly attributed to estrogen, which is an indispensable ingredient in nearly all contraceptives. For a long time these hormones had been related to carbohydrate metabolism, but the evaluation showed inconsistent results. For example, Nelson[12] and Nelson and Overholser[13] claimed that diabetic bitches and monkeys improved after taking estrogens, an observation that was, however, not confirmed.[22] Administering stilbestrol to rats under compulsory feeding, Ingle[10] and Ingle and Nezamis[11] found glycosuria in normal animals and increased glycosuria in animals with partial pancreatectomy. By means of a classic experiment Foglia Rodríguez, and their associates[5, 6, 16] observed a biphasic effect in castrated female rats with subtotal pancreatectomy that were receiving estrogens, specifically stilbestrol; elevation of blood sugar and glycosuria lasted for about a month, followed by a recovery period with normal blood sugar values. This protective secondary effect is associated with hyperplasia and hypertrophy of the islets of Langerhans and persists after suspension of treatment. Similar findings are seen in alloxan diabetes. It was difficult to apply these results obtained in laboratory animals to human beings without sufficiently controlled long-term studies.

Considering the increased use of contraceptives, we developed a research plan to investigate their possible side effects on glucose tolerance. From the start the 2 components of the pill, estrogen and progestin, were separately evaluated: the first group was composed of young women, but soon afterward we started a similar scheme in a group of climacteric women under estrogen therapy. Both groups are especially apt for our studies, since the patients not only undergo a prolonged treatment but also are willing to submit to periodic examinations, carried out every 3 months. Our first results have already been published.[3, 4, 15] In the meantime, we have followed a fair number of patients for more than 2 years. In this paper, which includes the total of our cases, we will describe our methods and the results in various therapy periods, and we will discuss the probable mechanism of the registered alterations.

Material and method

The principal aim of this study was to find the possible effects of estrogens and progestin which are employed in contraceptives, such as mestranol, ethinyl estradiol, chlormadinone, and norethisterone acetate, on carbohydrate metabolism. The evaluation was based on oral tolerance tests, either to simple glucose (GT) or combined with prednisone (PGT). Having been able to disregard the possible role of progestins 6 months after starting treatment,[4] we devoted our attention

Table I. Clinical histories related to diabetes

	202 young women	137 climacteric women
Family history:		
Positive	17	19
Negative	185	118
Obstetric findings:		
Large fetus	39	8
Others	22	7
Negative	127	119
Without data	14	3
Vulvovaginitis:		
Positive	14	18
Negative	175	114
Without data	13	5
Age at menarche:		
Under 11 years old	14	21
Over 11 years old	182	111
Without data	6	5

38

to the estrogens. To the women under study, we added a group of climacteric women with deprivation symptoms who had received estrogen therapy. Results before and during several treatment periods were compared.

Number of patients. A group of 339 women was clinically tested in the out patient clinics of Family Planning and Climacteric Disorders of the Department of Gynecology, and at the Section of Metabolic Diseases of the Department of Internal Medicine, University of Buenos Aires.

Age. There were 202 women between the ages of 19 and 40 years, and in the 137 climacteric women (41 to 55 years of age) we included 24 castrated patients.

Hormonal condition. Of the 202 women of reproductive age, 172 had previous ovulatory cycles, and 30 were nursing. The 112 climacteric women were subdivided in 68 pre- and 44 postmenopausal patients. Nine women had been surgically castrated for less than 1 year and 15 for more.

Histories related to diabetes. The clinical histories of all of the patients in this study with reference to diabetes are shown in Table I.

Drugs employed, method of administration, and dosage.

Mestranol. Mestranol (ethinyl estradiol 3-methyl ether was administered as a single agent in castrated and postmenopausal women in daily doses of 40 and 80 γ, either continuously or in periodic cycles of 15 to 20 days. In women of the reproductive age, sequential contraceptive therapy consisted of daily doses of 80 γ, combined with 2 mg. of chlormadinone during the last 3 to 5 days, or simultaneously with 5 mg. of norethisterone acetate per day. The women in this group, in whom we originally evaluated the possible influence of progestin, received later a sequential mestranol-chlormadinone regimen. All of these patients are designated as Group I (mestranol) since progestin did not modify their glucose tolerance.[4]

Norethisterone acetate (NEA). NEA was given as the single agent to 30 young women, most of them nursing, in daily doses of 5 mg. for 3 to 6 months.

Ethinyl estradiol (EE). A total of 52 young women were studied either with a sequential regimen of 100 γ per day, adding chlormadinone during the last 3 to 5 days, or with a combined treatment of 50 γ with 3 to 4 mg. norethisterone acetate per day.

1,3-Hydroxyethinyl estradiol diacetate. To 36 pre- and postmenopausal women this compound was administered at a rate of 25, 50, 75, and 100 γ per day, continuously or sequentially, combined with norethisterone acetate.

Estrone sulfate, dehydroequilin sulfate, and equilin sulfate. Daily doses of 2.5 mg. estrone sulfate and 0.5 mg. of the other agents were given to 40 climacteric women in a continuous or sequential regimen. Unfortunately the follow-up was too short to yield any definite conclusions.

Glucose tolerance test. Oral tolerance tests after previous administration of prednisone were performed before starting on the therapeutic program and later every 3 months. Many patients were controlled for more than 2 years. When abnormal PGT test values appeared at the first determination, GT tests were repeated to discard the possible influence of prednisone. We adopted the technique of Ruiz and associates.[17] After 3 days of a high-carbohydrate diet, 10 mg. of prednisone were given 8 and 2 hours before drawing a capillary blood sample. Immediately afterward, 100 Gm. of anhydrous glucose in a 20 per cent aqueous solution was administered, and blood samples drawn after 1, 2, and 3 hours. Blood was tested for its glucose content by the Somogyi-Nelson micromethod. Abnormal tests are those in which 3 of the 4 glucose determina-

Table II. Maximum normal values in a control series of tests

	Glucose tolerance test	Prednisone glucose tolerance test
Fasting	110	120
First hour	190	200
Second hour	140	150
Third hour	115	125

tions are above the maximum values of a control group, as shown in Table II.

Results

Group I. Mestranol. Table III shows the results related to the entire material in treatment periods of from 1 to 30 months. The daily doses were 40 to 80 γ. PGT tests yielded a higher proportion of abnormal results in the first and third months, and a lower one after the sixth. Toward the twelfth month the values were similar to controls prior to treatment and remained so for a 30 month follow-up. The statistical analysis re-

Table III. Prednisone glucose tolerance test in Group I—women taking mestranol (40 and 80 γ daily)

	No. of cases	Normal test	Abnormal test	Per cent of abnormal test	S.E.
Before treatment	125	117	8	6.4	±2.19
First and third months	86	37	49 (4)*	56.9	±5.34
Sixth month	27	17	10 (2)	37	±9.29
Ninth month	22	18	4 (4)	18.1	±8.20
Twelfth and fifteenth months	34	32	2	5.8	±4.01
Eighteenth and twenty-first months	32	31	1 (1)	3.1	±3.06
Twenty-fourth, twenty-seventh and thirtieth months	30	29	1	3.3	±3.26

*The figures in parentheses refer to patients in whom PGT test were found to be abnormal before starting medication (Tables III to VIII). Whenever these tests were abnormal prior to treatment, the alteration persisted in all examinations carried out during therapy.

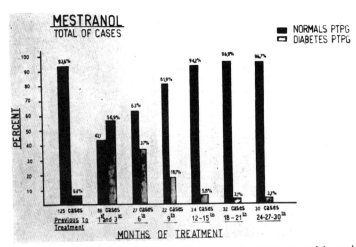

Fig. 1. Comparison of percentage of normal and abnormal responses to prednisone glucose tolerance test before and during treatment with mestranol in periods of from 1 to 30 months.

40

veals that the difference between the number of diabetic PGT tests before starting treatment and those registered after 1 and 3 months was very significant ($P < 0.0005$). Between the first, third, and sixth months it was also significant ($P < 0.05$), whereas the values found between the ninth and the thirtieth month lacked statistical significance.

In order to establish whether the differences might be related to their ages, the patients of Group I were divided into 2 subgroups, IA and IB (young and climacteric women). The partial results as seen in Tables IV and V show that the values obtained are similar to the results in the total of cases.

The apparent discrepancy between the number of patients with previous PGT tests and the 119 young women with mestranol

therapy was due to the fact that several are included as controls in the groups originally treated with NEA and EE. The difference between PGT tests before treatment and tests performed from the first to the third month was statistically very significant ($P < 0.0005$).

Although fewer cases were controlled in subgroup IB, the percentage of abnormal curves is similar to the ones of Subgroup IA. The differences between previous diabetic PGT test and the values registered between the first and third months were highly significant ($P < 0.0005$). Between the first and third months compared with the sixth to ninth month period they were significant ($P < 0.05$).

Group II. Norethisterone acetate. Table VI shows the results in Group II—the women taking norethisterone acetate. Since

Table IV. Prednisone glucose tolerance test in Subgroup IA—young women taking mestranol (80 γ daily)

	No. of cases	Normal	Abnormal	Per cent abnormal	S.E.
Before treatment	83	78	5	6	±2.61
First and third months	66	30	36 (2)	54.5	±6.13
Sixth month	24	15	9 (1)	37.5	±9.88
Ninth month	20	16	4 (1)	20	±8.94
Twelfth and fifteenth months	32	30	2	6.2	±4.26
Eighteenth and twenty-first months	31	30	1	3.2	±3.16
Twenty-fourth, twenty-seventh, and thirtieth months	29	28	1	3.4	±3.37

Table V. Prednisone glucose tolerance test in Subgroup IB—climacteric group taking mestranol (40 and 80 γ daily)

	No. of cases	Normal	Abnormal	Per cent abnormal	S.E.
Before treatment	42	39	13 (2)	7.1	±3.96
First and third months	20	7	3	65	±10.66
Sixth and ninth months	5	4	1 (1)	20	±17.89
More than 12 months	5	5	0		

41

the differences between previous PGT tests and the ones performed in various treatment periods (< 0.40 P < 0.30) were insignificant, most of the women were included in Groups I and III after the third month.

Group III. Ethinyl estradiol. Table VII shows the results related to all of the women taking EE either as a sequential regimen with chlormadinone or simultaneously combined with NEA, since these forms do not differ in their effect on glucose tolerance (Fig. 2). Statistical analysis shows that the difference between previous PGT tests and the tests performed in various treatment periods was not significant (< 0.45 P < 0.40).

Group IV. 1,3-Diacetate-6-hydroxyethinyl estradiol (SH-80-879). Table VIII summarizes the results in Group IV—the climacteric women taking 1,3-diacetate-6-hydroxyethinyl estradiol. The difference between previous PGT tests and tests in various treatment periods was not significant (< 0.40 P < 0.45).

Comment

In previous papers[3, 4, 15] we reported a decrease in glucose tolerance evidenced by a

Table VI. Prednisone glucose tolerance test in Group II—women taking norethisterone acetate (5 mg. daily)

	No. of cases	Normal	Abnormal	Per cent abnormal	S.E.
Before treatment	22	21	1	4.5	±4.42
First month	11	10	1	9	±8.63
Third month	16	15	1	6.2	±6.03
Sixth month	10	10	0		

Table VII. Prednisone glucose tolerance test in Group III—women taking ethinyl estradiol (50 and 100 γ daily)

	No. of cases	Normal	Abnormal	Per cent abnormal	S.E.
Before treatment	48	45	3	6.2	±3.48
First and third months	26	24	2	7.6	±5.20
Sixth and ninth months	23	22	1	4.3	±4.23
Twelfth, fifteenth, eighteenth, and twenty-fourth months	13	12	1	7.2	±7.17

Table VIII. Prednisone glucose tolerance tests in Group IV—women taking 1,3-diacetate-6-hydroxy ethinyl estradiol (25, 50, 75, and 100 γ daily)

	No. of cases	Normal	Abnormal	Per cent abnormal	S.E.
Before treatment	36	33	3	8.3	±4.59
First month	21	19	2 (2)	9.5	±6.39
Third and sixth months	19	16	3 (2)	15.7	±8.34

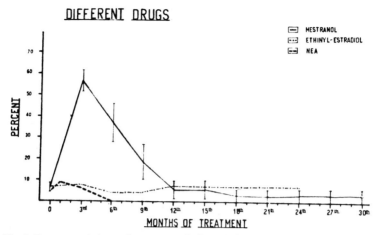

DIFFERENT DRUGS

☐ MESTRANOL
☐ ETHINYL-ESTRADIOL
☐ NEA

MONTHS OF TREATMENT

Fig. 2. Percentage of abnormal responses to PGT test before and during various periods of treatment with mestranol, norethisterone acetate, and ethinyl estradiol.

higher frequency of abnormal PGT tests after the first month of therapy in women taking mestranol. At the same time it became clear that this effect was not due to norsteroids and progestins or to ethinyl estradiol, currently employed in contraceptive treatment. The percentage of abnormal PGT tests was higher in women with diabetic family histories and early menarche. This finding implied an important practical consequence, since mestranol is utilized in many other conditions wherein long-term replacement estrogen therapy is indicated. Although it is a significant alteration, we observed a decreasing tendency when treatment was continued for more than 9 months. We decided therefore to pursue the research for a period of 2 years or more, increasing the number of mestranol-treated women and trying out other estrogens as well.

The data obtained in a larger group of women confirm our previous findings, which showed that mestranol is the drug responsible for decreases in glucose tolerance during the first 9 months of therapy when daily doses of 40 and 80 γ are given. No modifications of PGT tests were observed when the patients received 20 γ per day or when

ethinyl estradiol or ethinyl estradiol diacetate was administered.[4] There was no difference in glucose tolerance between the women of different ages in their reproductive years and in the climacteric. The most interesting finding, however, was the fact that a prolonged follow-up allowed us to prove that the effect on carbohydrate metabolism was only transient, since the percentage of abnormal PGT tests decreased after 9 months and reached normal levels after 12 (Fig. 3). These normal levels have been recorded also in 30 women evaluated for a 30 month period.

The significance of decrease in glucose tolerance is hard to explain, but we feel that it is an expression of subclinical diabetes since its highest frequency is observed in women with family histories of diabetes and early menarche. Furthermore Spellacy and Carlson[18] and Spellacy, Carlson, and Birk[19] reported an elevation of plasma insulin levels similar to the findings in the early stages of diabetes in women taking oral contraceptives containing mestranol.

Analysis of the clinical and experimental information we have gathered allows us to compare our data with the conclusions of

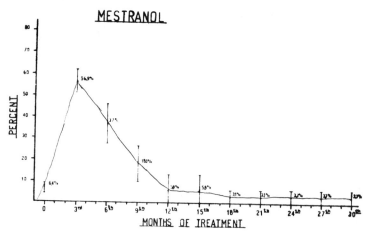

Fig. 3. Incidence of abnormal PGT before and during various periods of treatment with mestranol.

Foglia in his previously mentioned paper on experimental diabetes, which apparently did not coincide with our first results. By following patients for more than one year, we have confirmed in women the "biphasic effect" which those authors had described in rats; in other words, a recovery of glucose tolerance which, according to their findings, is due to hypertrophy and hyperplasia of pancreatic islets. The higher insulinemia values[4] support this interpretation. We feel, however, that control should be continued for still longer periods and that insulin assays should be repeated periodically not only in fasting conditions but also in tolerance curves. We have started on a similar program although we are aware of the difficult interpretation of the complex and not yet fully understood homeostatic mechanism of plasma insulin.

The preceding comments refer to the adaptation period of the organism but do not explain the lowering of glucose tolerance during the first months. Frantz and Rabkin[7] stimulated the liberation of growth hormone (HGH) with its known diabetogenic effect,[9] employing stilbestrol. They also found that mestranol and norethynodrel administration is followed by a remarkable elevation of HGH, which therefore might be held responsible for the lowered glucose tolerance in the first months of treatment. The increase of nonesterificated fatty acids seen by Wynn and Doar[21] in contraceptive therapy containing mestranol support this interpretation. The significance of these findings however remains to be determined.

After the first alarm caused by the confirmed lowering of glucose tolerance during the first months of therapy, the subsequent recovery seems to favor continuation of contraceptive treatment with pills containing mestranol. However, this recovery, undoubtedly due to an adaption of the organism, will have to be attentively considered with all of its possible consequences. Since the normalization of tests is probably caused by pancreatic stimulation, and since these treatments usually continue for long periods of time, the question arises as to whether after several years exhaustion of the pancreatic islets with all its foreseen consequences might not have to be feared. On the other hand there is the question of whether these alterations are reversible or not. To solve these problems it will be neces-

44

sary to repeat experiments in rats using, specifically, mestranol, and to continue observations of patients for several years. In another group, tests should be repeated after having suspended treatment. These would be the means of obtaining adequate information about the risks which a prolonged administration of mestranol might entail. In the meantime it would be wise for women with latent diabetes or with family or personal histories of the disease to avoid its use.

We are indebted to Prof. F. Toranzo for his statistical analysis of the data and to Mrs. Ellen Kundegraber for preparing the manuscript.

REFERENCES

1. Buchler, D., and Warren, J. C.: AMER. J. OBSTET. GYNEC. 95: 479, 1966.
2. Collip. J. B., Selye, H., and Neufeld, A.: Amer. J. Physiol. 119: 289, 1937.
3. Di Paola, G., Puchulu, F., Robín, M., Nicholson, R., and Marti, M. L.: Lancet 1: 1163, 1967.
4. Di Paola, G., Puchulu, F., Robín, M., Nicholson, R., and Marti, M. L.: AMER. J. OBSTET. GYNEC. 101: 206, 1968.
5. Foglia, V. G.: Rev. Soc. Argent. Biol. 20: 21, 1944.
6. Foglia, V. G., Rodríguez, R. L., and Schuster, N.: Rev. Soc. Argent. Biol. 23: 202, 1947.
7. Frantz, A. G., and Rabkin, M. T.: J. Clin. Endocr. 25: 1470, 1965.
8. Gerschberg, H., Javier, Z., and Hulse, M.: Diabetes 13: 378, 1964.
9. Houssay, B. A., and Biasotti, A.: Rev. Soc. Argent. Biol. 6: 8, 1930.
10. Ingle, D. J.: Endocrinology 29: 839, 1941.
11. Ingle, D. J., and Nezamis, J. E.: Endocrinology 33: 181, 1943.
12. Nelson, W. O.: Endocrinology 19: 187, 1935.
13. Nelson, W. O., and Overholser, M.: Endocrinology 20: 437, 1936.
14. Posner, M. A., Silvertone, F. A., Pomerance, W., and Nechama, S.: Obstet. Gynec. 29: 87, 1967.
15. Puchulu, F., Di Paola, G. M. L., Robín, M., Nicholson, R., and Groppa, G.: Sixth Congress Int. Diabetes Fed., 1967, p. 122.
16. Rodríguez, R. R.: Fifth Congress Int. Diabetes Fed., 1965, p. 288.
17. Ruiz, M., Puchulu, F. E., Busquet, I., and Busquet, I. C.: Prensa Méd. Argent. 51: 169, 1967.
18. Spellacy, W. E., and Carlson, K. L.: AMER. J. OBSTET. GYNEC. 95: 475, 1966.
19. Spellacy, W. E., Carlson, K. L., and Birk, S. A.: Diabetes 16: 590, 1967.
20. Spellacy, W. E., Carlson, K. L., and Schade, S. L.: J. A. M. A. 202: 451, 1967.
21. Wynn, V., and Doar, J. W.: Lancet 2: 714, 1966.
22. Young, F. G.: Lancet 1: 600, 1941.

Vitamin B_6 metabolism in users of oral contraceptive agents. I. Abnormal urinary xanthurenic acid excretion and its correction by pyridoxine[1,2]

A. Leonard Luhby,[3] M.D., Myron Brin,[4] Ph.D., Myron Gordon,[5] M.D., Patricia Davis,[6] R.N., Maureen Murphy,[6] R.N., and Herbert Spiegel,[7] Ph.D.

Women using oral contraceptive agents containing estrogen analogues (OCA) have been reported to excrete an increased amount of metabolic intermediates of the tryptophan–niacin pathway. This occurs spontaneously (1) as well as after tryptophan metabolic loading (2). The abnormality has been attributed to a "relative" vitamin B_6 deficiency presumably induced by the estrogenic steroids (2, 3). Administration of large oral doses of pyridoxine hydrochloride reduced the increased urinary excretion of tryptophan metabolites in individuals taking an OCA (4–6).

Although the clinical consequences of this altered vitamin B_6 metabolism in the tryptophan metabolic pathway have not been fully elucidated, it is of interest that the depression, mood, and sleep pattern changes encountered in a significant number of OCA-using women (7–9) may be alleviated by a daily oral dose of 50 mg pyridoxine hydrochloride (8); in many, 25 mg daily was ineffective (F. Winston, personal communication).

Because of the clinical effectiveness and acceptability of the hormonal contraceptives there is considerable interest in correcting, if possible, the metabolic derangements resulting from their use (10). A systematic study was therefore undertaken to determine the minimum daily oral dose of pyridoxine hydrochloride necessary to normalize the urinary excretion of tryptophan metabolites following an oral tryptophan load in women using OCA.

Abnormal tryptophan metabolism, as measured by excessive urinary excretion of xanthurenic acid (XA) after a tryptophan load, was revealed in about three-quarters of the women tested. A daily oral dose of 25 mg pyridoxine hydrochloride was found to be necessary to normalize the urinary excretion of XA in all subjects. A preliminary report of this work has appeared (11).

The effect of OCA administration upon the urinary excretion of other tryptophan metabolites and their correction by pyridoxine will be presented in a separate report.

Materials and Methods

Clinical subjects

Forty-three female subjects participated in the study. They ranged in age from 21 to 42 years, averaging 27.8. All were nurses, secretaries, or other hospital workers, and all were in good health. Two subjects with sickle-cell–hemoglobin C disease had hemoglobin levels of 10 g/100 ml, lived a fairly normal life, and had given birth to one or more children. None of the participants took any medications during the study period other than those noted below.

Thirty-three subjects had been taking an oral contraceptive agent for periods ranging from 3 months to 6 years. Ten participants were not using these medications.

Oral contraceptive agents

These included Ovulen, five subjects; Ovral, six; Norinyl-1, one; Norlestrin, two; Ortho-Novum-1,

[2] Supported in part by a grant-in-aid from the National Vitamin Foundation.

46

TABLE 1
Type and content of estrogen and progestogen analogues in oral contraceptive agents

Trade name	Estrogen	µg/tablet	Progestogen	mg/tablet
Norinyl-1[a]	Mestranol	50	Norethindrone	1
Ortho-Novum-1[b]	Mestranol	50	Norethindrone	1
C-Quens[c]	Mestranol	80	Chlormadinone acetate	1
Ortho-Novum 1/80[b]	Mestranol	80	Norethindrone	1
Ortho-Novum-2[b]	Mestranol	100	Norethindrone	2
Ovulen 21[d]	Mestranol	100	Ethynodiol diacetate	1
Norlestrin[e]	Ethinyl estradiol	50	Norethindrone acetate	1
Ovral[f]	Ethinyl estradiol	50	Norgestrel	0.5
Oracon[g]	Ethinyl estradiol	100	Dimethisterone	25

[a] Syntex Laboratories Inc., Palo Alto, California. [b] Ortho Pharmaceutical Corp., Raritan, New Jersey. [c] Eli Lilly and Co., Indianapolis, Indiana. [d] G. D. Searle and Co., Chicago, Illinois. [e] Parke, Davis and Co., Detroit, Michigan. [f] Wyeth Labs., Division American Home Products Corp., Philadelphia, Pa. [g] Mead Johnson and Co., Evansville, Indiana.

four; Ortho-Novum-2, ten; Ortho-Novum 1/80, one; Oracon, two; and C-Quens, two. The type and content of the estrogen and progestogen analogue in each are shown in Table 1.

Experimental design and methodology

Each subject was followed through three consecutive menstrual cycles during which the following experimental plan was carried out:

Tryptophan loading. A 2-g L-tryptophan metabolic load was administered orally in 6 to 8 oz milk to each of the OCA users just before the start, in the middle, and just before the end of the contraceptive pill regimen. The 10 control subjects (non-OCA users) were loaded 5 days after the onset of the last menses, in the middle of the following cycle, and just before the start of the next menses in order to evaluate the hormonal effects of a normal menstrual cycle upon the xanthurenic acid excretion. There were thus at least nine tryptophan loading periods for each participant. In a few subjects, a load test was done prior to the start of the experimental plan.

The 2-g, rather than a 5- or 10-g, L-tryptophan load was chosen because reports (12, 13) indicated that this loading dose was least likely to distort the metabolic state through overloading or a substrate induction of the enzymes (13) in the tryptophan–niacin pathway. The 2-g dose also has been reported to give the greatest reproducibility of the amount of tryptophan metabolic intermediates excreted in the urine after metabolic loading (14).

Urine xanthurenic acid. Urine to be assayed for its XA content was collected in acid for an 8-hr period after the tryptophan load. This interval permitted the subject to complete the collection during her work hours at the hospital. Acidification with 6 N HCl to bring the final pH to 1 to 2 permitted storage of the urine at room temperature without deterioration of the tryptophan metabolites until assayed.

To compare the uniformity of the XA excretion after tryptophan in the 8-hr urine collection used here with that of the 24-hr collection employed by

others, fractional urine collections were obtained in four subjects using OCA.

The creatinine content of each urine collection was determined as an index of the completeness of the 8-hr sample.

Urine XA was determined by a modification of the manual Wachstein and Gudaitis assay (15), as adapted to an autoanalyzer technique by Nowak and Körner (16). Results were expressed as micromoles XA per 8-hr urine excretion. Values obtained by the Nowak and Körner automated assay were virtually identical with those obtained by the manual method. The assay has a sensitivity of 0.05 µmole/ml urine (16).

Pyridoxine administration. Pyridoxine hydrochloride in tablet form was administered orally simultaneously with the "pill" in daily doses of 2 and 5 mg during the first and third OCA cycles, respectively, to one group and to another group, 10 or 20 mg during these same times. A placebo (lactose) was administered in the same manner during the second cycle to establish a nonpyridoxine supplemented control period for each participant. When the OCA was discontinued at the completion of a 20- or 21-day course, the pyridoxine or placebo was also discontinued. In each case, the OCA was taken in the manner previously used by the participant. The pyridoxine and placebo tablets were coded so that the subject did not know their content or the experimental plan. Five OCA users were followed for three cycles without pyridoxine as "positive" controls, as were eight of the ten non-OCA users, as "negative" controls.

Results

Comparison of 8- and 24-hour urine collection periods for xanthurenic acid excretion

In Fig. 1 are presented the results of these experiments in tabular and graphic form. The average 8-hr urinary XA excretion in the four patients, 88 μmoles, represented 63.4% of 139.1 μmoles, the average 24-hr excretion. From the line graph, it can be seen that the 8-hr excretion was approximately the same fraction of the 24-hr excretion in each of the study subjects. Thus the 8-hr urine XA excretion after a 2-g L-tryptophan load can be expected to provide a constant fraction of that excreted in 24 hr.

Urine xanthurenic acid excretion after 2 g L-tryptophan in normal non-OCA using women

The xanthurenic acid excretion values for the eight to ten loading tests performed as outlined in eight non-OCA-using subjects during three menstrual cycles are plotted in Fig. 2A. For the individual women, the mean XA excretion for all the tests performed on each, ranged from 9.2 ± 4.9 to 18.3 ± 5.3 μmoles/8 hr (Table 2). In none of the women studied was there a consistent midmenstrual cycle increase of the xanthurenic acid excretion after the 2-g L-tryptophan load. The

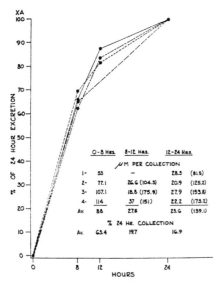

FIG. 1. The 24-hr fractional urinary xanthurenic acid excretion values following a 2-g L-tryptophan (oral) metabolic load, given to four women using an OCA. Values in parentheses represent the cumulative amounts.

TABLE 2

Average urinary xanthurenic acid excretion following a 2-g L-tryptophan metabolic load[a, b]

Normal non-OCA using women	OCA-using women
9.2 ± 4.9	41.86 ± 32.6
11.3 ± 7.6	63.9 ± 46.2
14.0 ± 5.5	78.7 ± 53.8
14.6 ± 6.6	210.1 ± 102.5
15.2 ± 6.3	275.8 ± 153.7
16.5 ± 5.2	
16.6 ± 7.0	
18.3 ± 5.3	
Range: undetectable to 32.1	9.4 to 553.0

[a] 8 to 10 individual loading tests per subject.
[b] Urinary xanthurenic acid output micromoles/8 hr ± 1 SD.

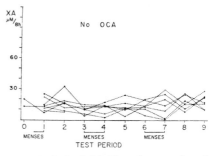

FIG. 2. A, B. Serial 8-hr urinary xanthurenic acid excretion values following repeat 2-g L-tryptophan (oral) metabolic loading during three consecutive menstrual cycles: A) in eight normal women not taking an oral contraceptive agent (OCA) and B) in five women using an OCA. Test period "0" represents a preexperimental period test in the latter half of the preceding menstrual cycle.

FIG. 2A. For women not taking an OCA: test period 1 is 5 days after the onset of the last menses; 2 is midmenstrual and 3 is 1 to 2 days prior to the onset of the next menses. Periods 4, 5, 6 and 7, 8, 9 are the corresponding times of the next two natural menstrual cycles.

graphic plot of the data (Fig. 2A) shows a remarkable uniformity of excretion values in non-OCA using women after repeat loads performed over an extended period of time. Because none of the non-OCA using women excreted more than 35 μmoles xanthurenic acid, at any of the test times, excretions greater than 35 μmoles/8 hr were considered

48

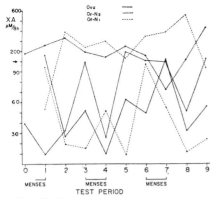

FIG. 2B. For women taking an OCA: test period 1 is the day prior to the start of the next OCA regimen; 2 is mid-OCA regimen and 3 is 1 to 2 days prior to its termination. Periods 4, 5, 6 and 7, 8, 9 are the corresponding times of the next two OCA-menstrual cycles. No OCA was taken between periods 3 to 4 and 6 to 7.

Ovu = Ovulen-21 containing 100 μg estrogen analogue; Or-N2 = Ortho-Novum-2, 100 μg and Or-N-1 = Ortho-Novum-1, 50 μg estrogen analogue/tablet.

to be abnormally increased under the test conditions.

Urine xanthurenic acid excretion after 2 g L-tryptophan in OCA-using women

The XA excretion after a tryptophan load varied over a much larger range in OCA using women (Fig. 2B) than in the non-OCA using control subjects (Fig. 2A). Among the five participants who were followed for three "menstrual cycles" without pyridoxine supplementation, the range of excretion values for any single load test was 9.4 to 553 μmoles/8 hr. The average excretion for the nine loading tests in individual subjects is given in Table 2.

Among the total group of 33 OCA using participants, the maximum excretion during any of the tryptophan loading tests ranged from 20 to 663 μmoles/8 hr, with an average of 167.5 μmoles. Approximately three-quarters of the women using an OCA excreted more than 35 μmoles urinary xanthurenic acid pᵣr 8 hr during one or more of the test periods (Fig. 3). Thus, about twenty-five percent of the subjects were "non-reactors"

to the oral contraceptive agent after the 2-g load.

Because the two analogues, mestranol and ethinyl estradiol, in the oral contraceptive agents used by the participants in the study do not have the same estrogenic activity (17), an attempt was made to evaluate their relative effect on the urinary excretion of XA by plotting the maximum excretion of each participant during any test period against the dose of the estrogen analogue in the OCA employed. These data are shown in Fig. 3. It was noted that the average of the maximum XA excretion for individuals taking 50 μg mestranol was 222.4 μmoles, whereas those taking 50 μg ethinyl estradiol had an average maximum excretion of 71.25 μmoles under the same conditions. The comparable values for 100 μg mestranol and ethinyl estradiol were 192.5 and 170.5 μmoles, respectively. Although the number of values at some dose levels are not ade-

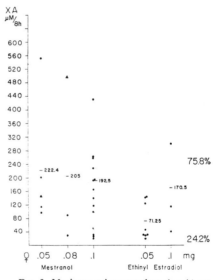

FIG. 3. Maximum urinary xanthurenic acid output values following a 2-g L-tryptophan (oral) load of 33 subjects using an OCA, plotted against the type and amount of estrogen analogue employed in the oral contraceptive medication used. The triangular shaped points are the values for the two subjects with sickle-cell–hemoglobin C disease.

49

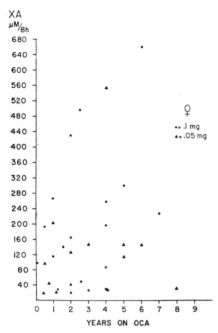

XA
$\mu M/8h$

680
640
600
560
520
480   ♀
440   •• .1 mg
400   ▲▪ .05 mg
360
320
280
240
200
160
120
80
40

0 1 2 3 4 5 6 7 8 9
YEARS ON OCA

FIG. 4. Maximum urinary xanthurenic acid excretion values following a 2-g L-tryptophan (oral) load of 33 subjects plotted against the number of years each used an OCA continuously.

quate for statistical comparison, the trend appears to be for lower excretions of XA to occur after 50 μg ethinyl estradiol as compared with the same dose of mestranol. This did not appear to apply at the 100 μg dose level of each.

The maximum XA excretions for the two subjects with sickle-cell–hemoglobin C disease were 145 and 496 μmoles. Although only two subjects with this disorder were evaluated, their excretions at other times and their responses to pyridoxine did not appear to be greatly different from the other participants.

In Fig. 4, the maximum xanthurenic acid excretion value is plotted against the number of years the subject continuously used an OCA. Continued use of the pill did not appear to result in a decrease of its effect in producing an increase in the urinary excretion of XA. In fact, the trend appears to

be towards increasing values with longer use.

Response of the increased xanthurenic aciduria to vitamin B_6

The response of the 18 OCA using women with increased xanthurenic aciduria to vitamin B_6 at four dosage levels is shown in Fig. 5A, B, C.

It is apparent from inspection of Fig. 5A that, whereas the 2-mg dose of vitamin B_6 partially corrected only a small percentage of the subjects tested, and the 5-mg dose was more effective, neither dose level could be considered uniformly effective. However, although the 10-mg level normalized 75% of the subjects by the end of the OCA regimen (Table 3), 14% remained incompletely corrected at the 20-mg dosage level.

The dose–response data are summarized in Table 3. The number and percentage of subjects at each dose level who failed to re-

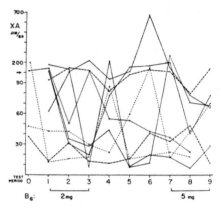

XA
$\mu M/8h$

700
200
90
60
30

TEST PERIOD 0 1 2 3 4 5 6 7 8 9

B_6:   2 mg   5 mg

FIG. 5A

FIG. 5A to C. Effect of pyridoxine hydrochloride upon the xanthurenic aciduria after 2-g L-tryptophan load in 18 women using an OCA and exhibiting abnormally increased urinary xanthurenic acid.

The test period legend is the same as for Fig. 2B. Following a pre-course load (test periods 1 and 7) pyridoxine hydrochloride in dosage shown was given with the pill throughout its course. The middle OCA course (test periods 4, 5, and 6) acted as a nonpyridoxine control period during which a placebo was given with the OCA.

Arrow on ordinate: point at which scale for xanthurenic acid changes from 10 to 100 μmoles per division.

50

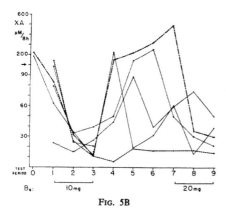

Fig. 5B

spond were examined in an attempt to identify the dose of pyridoxine hydrochloride that could be expected to correct the increased xanthurenic aciduria after the 2-g L-tryptophan load in "all" individuals on OCA who were "reactive", i.e., those who reacted to the OCA with an increased urinary XA excretion. The regression analysis of the dose–response data revealed that an oral dose of 25 mg pyridoxine hydrochloride would be the minimum amount necessary to normalize the increased xanthurenic aciduria of "all" reactive women using an OCA.

Discussion

The results of this study present new data in several areas concerning the influence of OCA use on vitamin B_6 and tryptophan metabolism.

OCA use and urinary xanthurenic acid

Rose (2) and Price et al. (4) previously reported that women using oral contraceptive medications excreted an increased amount of urinary xanthurenic acid after a tryptophan metabolic load. The present study demonstrated that after a 2-g tryptophan load about 75% of the women using an OCA have this disturbance of tryptophan metabolism, whereas in the remaining 25%, the OCA did not have this influence. It is of interest that in reactive women, the effect of the OCA was relatively rapid, often rising sharply soon after commencement of the medication and decreasing strikingly in

many women during the menses interval when no OCA was taken. In addition, this responsiveness did not decrease with continued long-term use of the OCA. Women using OCA up to 6 years continued to manifest this abnormality of amino acid metabolism. It was also of interest that the XA output in reactive women using an OCA containing 50 μg ethinyl estradiol was considerably less than that of women taking the same dose of mestranol. This finding may aid in the future choice of estrogen analogues for OCA use.

Tryptophan metabolic loading to augment urinary xanthurenic acid

Although a 10-g DL-tryptophan metabolic loading dose was generally employed for the average adult in early studies, the induction effect of this substrate on a key

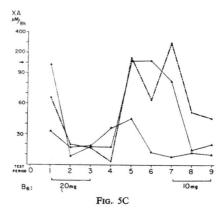

Fig. 5C

TABLE 3

Response to vitamin B_6 of the increased xanthurenic aciduria resulting from OCA use

Dose as pyridoxine hydrochloride, mg	Number of evaluatable trials[a]	Number without effect	Percent without effect
2	10	9	90.
5	9	4	33.3
10	8	2	25.
20	7	1	14.3

[a] A trial was considered to be evaluatable if the change in the XA excretion at the middle and end of the OCA cycle was in the same direction.

enzyme system, tryptophan oxygenase, in the metabolic pathway being tested (13), resulted in the employment of smaller doses in order to minimize this effect. Currently, the consensus is that a 2-g L-tryptophan load will produce a significant increase of the urinary XA in vitamin B_6 metabolic disturbances of clinical importance and not result in a spuriously elevated excretion (14). The difference in effect of a 2- and 5-g loading dose is illustrated by our failure to consistently find a midmenstrual increase of the urinary XA excretion after a 2-g L-tryptophan load in normal non-OCA using women. This confirms similar findings by Price et al. (18) who also employed a 2-g L-tryptophan metabolic load. On the other hand, several workers using a 5-g L-tryptophan load (19, 20) found a midmenstrual increase in urinary XA excretion, implying that a relative vitamin B_6 deficiency existed at mid-cycle.

To our knowledge there have been no previous studies in which the urinary XA excretion was measured after repeat tryptophan metabolic loads were administered to the same individual over a 3-month period. The relative constancy of the level of excretion upon repeating the metabolic challenge in the non-OCA using normals (Fig. 2A) contrasts strikingly with the greater variability of excretion after repeat loads in many OCA users (Fig. 2B). Also documented in these studies is the validity of the 8-hr versus the 24-hr urinary collection for these purposes. The convenience of the shorter collection period may be of crucial practical importance for clinical studies in non-hospitalized individuals. Employing a 2-g L-tryphophan load and an 8-hr urine collection, the normal adult female apparently excretes less than 35 μmoles XA.

Relationship of increased xanthurenic aciduria to vitamin B_6 deficiency

The demonstration by Lepkovsky and his colleagues in 1943 (21) that xanthurenic acid, a compound derived from dietary tryptophan, was excreted in increased amounts in experimental nutritional vitamin B_6 deficiency in rats, established increased xanthurenic aciduria as an index of vitamin B_6

deficiency. In experimental nutritional vitamin B_6 deficiency in man, however, it has been found necessary to administer a tryptophan metabolic load to demonstrate the vitamin B_6 inadequacy via an increased urinary XA excretion (22). The mechanism by which this increased XA occurs in vitamin B_6 deficiency states, however, has not yet been completely explained. Increased urinary XA excretion after a tryptophan load has also been observed in a variety of clinical conditions such as rheumatoid arthritis (23), infection (24), and pregnancy (25), in which the classical clinical manifestations of human nutritional vitamin B_6 deficiency, i.e., dermatitis, peripheral neuritis, and vitamin B_6-responsive anemia, are generally absent. The significance of the increased XA excretion as it relates to a vitamin B_6 deficiency state in the latter conditions has been only partially resolved.

Administration of estrogenic steroids and their analogues also results in an increased xanthurenic aciduria. In animal systems, these steroids have been shown to cause two major alterations in vitamin B_6–tryptophan metabolism: *1)* an increase of hepatic tryptophan oxygenase activity (3, 26, 27), which results in the sending of more tryptophan down the pathway to niacin and accounts in great measure for the increased production of a variety of the metabolites of this pathway; and *2)* a reduction in the affinity for pyridoxal phosphate of two of the vitamin B_6-dependent enzymes of tryptophan metabolism, kynureninase and kynurenine transaminase (28). The increased traffic of tryptophan metabolites down the pathway due to the increased oxygenase activity combined with the reduced kynureninase activity, particularly that concerned with the conversion of 3-hydroxykynurenine to 3-hydroxyanthranilic acid, apparently overwhelms the functional capacity of the latter enzyme system. This results in an accumulation of preceding metabolites including XA. This "functional vitamin B_6 deficiency" state, somewhat akin to a "vitamin B_6-dependency," is believed to occur in women who use an OCA containing an estrogen analogue, since large doses of pyridoxine administered to such women will normalize the urinary excretion of XA.

52

Clinical significance of estrogen-altered tryptophan metabolism

The clinical significance in the human of this alteration of tryptophan metabolism and the resulting increased body burden of tryptophan metabolic intermediates has yet to be satisfactorily elucidated. In animal systems, tryptophan metabolites have been shown to interfere with gluconeogenesis (29), oxidative phosphorylation (30), insulin metabolism resulting in diabetes (31), and to be carcinogenic when implanted into the urinary bladder of mice (32, 33). These effects were all detrimental and suggest that these metabolites are undesirable.

Although there were no classical clinical manifestations of vitamin B_6 deficiency in the reactive OCA-using women in this study, it has been suggested recently, that depression, mood, and sleep pattern changes encountered in OCA users (7–9) may be related to the abnormal tryptophan metabolism resulting from OCA use through a reduction in brain serotonin (5-hydroxytryptamine) (34). The evidence for a decrease in brain serotonin as the cause for depression syndromes in man is meager (35), but there is a rationale for suspecting that such a mechanism may occur in the depression associated with OCA use, since serotonin arises from tryptophan, and a B_6-dependent enzyme step is required for its formation from the latter. The shunting of tryptophan down the niacin pathway as a result of the use of OCA containing an estrogen analogue may significantly reduce the tryptophan available for serotonin production (34). Interference with the pyridoxal phosphate requiring decarboxylation reaction of 5-hydroxytryptophan (the immediate precursor of serotonin) by estrogen conjugates (28), as well as interference with serotonin formation by tryptophan metabolic intermediates (34), has been reported in animal systems. In this connection, the report of the alleviation of depression symptoms in OCA users by a daily oral dose of 50 mg pyridoxine hydrochloride (8) is intriguing and warrants confirmation.

Amount of vitamin B_6 required to correct OCA-altered tryptophan metabolism

These studies concerning the amount of vitamin B_6, as pyridoxine hydrochloride, required to normalize the increased urinary excretion of tryptophan metabolites after a 2-g L-tryptophan load in OCA users were prompted by the above reports as well as by the current interest in correcting metabolic abnormalities resulting from OCA use (10). This was the first systematic attempt to obtain dose–response data for the correction of this abnormality when the vitamin is administered with the pill for a 20- or 21-day period. The extrapolated dose level of 25 mg is clearly considerably above the best estimates of the amount ingested daily in the average American diet, which is about 1 mg (36). It is also much higher than the 2-mg Recommended Dietary Allowance (RDA) for vitamin B_6 in the United States (37) and the United Kingdom (38).

Because the 25-mg value was extrapolated from a dose–response curve, it is suggested that a safety factor should be incorporated, as is the case in establishing an RDA (37), and that a level of 30 mg pyridoxine hydrochloride daily be recommended for OCA users to normalize the increased urinary tryptophan metabolite excretion.

There are approximately 7 to 8 million women in the United States alone who currently use an OCA. Since this study indicates that a great majority of OCA users have abnormal tryptophan metabolism, we are faced with a readily correctable metabolic abnormality in a large segment of an otherwise relatively healthy and young population. Furthermore, the metabolic abnormality appears to continue throughout the period of OCA use. For some, this may be in excess of 15 to 20 years. In view of the emerging evidence that abnormal tryptophan metabolism and the intermediary metabolites thereby produced may be detrimental, it would appear desirable to supplement the dietary vitamin B_6 intake of OCA users with pyridoxine hydrochloride.

Summary

The response of the increased urinary xanthurenic acid (XA) excretion following a 2-g L-tryptophan load to oral doses of 2, 5, 10, and 20 mg pyridoxine hydrochloride was systematically studied in a group of women using oral contraceptive agents (OCA). This was done through three consecutive menstrual cycles in each subject. Vitamin B_6

was given during the first and third cycles, whereas the middle cycle was a nonvitamin B_6-supplemented control (placebo) period. Tryptophan load tests were done at the beginning, in the middle, and at the end of each menstrual cycle. None of 10 non-OCA using control subjects excreted over 35 μmoles XA/8 hr. The majority of OCA users excreted in excess of this amount with an average of 167 μmoles. Those with increased XA excretion, positive reactors, comprised 75% of the OCA using group.

The 8-hr urine collection period was found to contain a relatively constant fraction (average, 63.4%) of the 24-hr xanthurenic acid excretion after a 2-g L-tryptophan oral load. As such, it was a valid and reliable urine collection period for this index of vitamin B_6 inadequacy.

Detrimental metabolic effects of various tryptophan metabolites in animal systems, interference with gluconeogenesis, oxidative phosphorylation, insulin metabolism, and in being carcinogenic, were pointed out.

The 2-mg dose of pyridoxine hydroxychloride, equivalent to the Recommended Dietary Allowance (37, 38) of vitamin B_6, was sufficient to correct only 10% of the women studied, whereas the 20-mg dose did not correct all subjects. A regression analysis of the dose–response data revealed that 25 mg would be required to correct all OCA using women. In view of the limited number of subjects studied, a dose of 30 mg (allowing 5 mg as a safety factor) is recommended to correct the altered vitamin B_6-tryptophan metabolism resulting from OCA use. ▨

We are indebted to Mr. H. T. T. Chang, Department of Research Statistics, Hoffmann-La Roche, Inc., for the regression analysis of the dose–response data, to Sara Kossowsky, R.N., M.A., for assistance in setting up administrative aspects of the study, to Robert L. Naylor, B.S., Maryse Sambour and Josephine Quichiz, M.A., for technical assistance, and Herbert Rich, M.A., Statistician, Department of Pediatrics, New York Medical College, for assistance with some of the statistical analysis of the data.

References

1. TOSELAND, P. A., AND S. PRICE. Tryptophan and oral contraceptives. *Brit. Med. J.* 1: 777, 1969.

2. ROSE, D. P. Excretion of xanthurenic acid in the urine of women taking progestogen-oestrogen preparations. *Nature* 210: 196, 1966.

3. BRIN, M. Pyridoxine, estrogenic contraceptive steroids (ECS) and tryptophan metabolism. *Federation Proc.* 29: 824, 1970.

4. PRICE, J. M., M. J. THORNTON AND L. M. MUELLER. Tryptophan metabolism in women using steroid hormones for ovulation control. *Am. J. Clin. Nutr.* 20: 452, 1967.

5. BROWN, R. R., D. P. ROSE, J. M. PRICE AND H. WOLF. Tryptophan metabolism as affected by anovulatory agents. *Ann. N. Y. Acad. Sci.* 166: 44, 1969.

6. ROSE, D. P. The influence of oestrogens on tryptophan metabolism in man. *Clin. Sci.* 31: 265, 1966.

7. KAYE, B. M. Oral contraceptives and depression. *J. Am. Med. Assoc.* 186: 522, 1963.

8. BAUMBLATT, M. J., AND F. WINSTON. Pyridoxine and the pill. *Lancet* 1: 832, 1970.

9. HERZBERG, B. N., A. L. JOHNSON AND S. BROWN. Depressive symptoms and oral contraceptives. *Brit. Med. J.* 4: 142, 1970.

10. SCHROGIE, J. J. Oral contraceptives: a status report. *Food Drug Admin. Papers.* Washington D. C.: U. S. Govt. Printing Office, May 1970, p. 23.

11. LUHBY, A. L., P. DAVIS, M. MURPHY, M. GORDON, M. BRIN AND H. SPIEGEL. Pyridoxine and oral contraceptives. *Lancet* 2: 1083, 1970.

12. COURSIN, D. B. Recommendations for standardization of the tryptophan load test. *Am. J. Clin. Nutr.* 14: 56, 1964.

13. KNOX, W. E. Adaptative enzymes in the regulation of animal metabolism. In: *Physiological Adaptation.* Washington D. C.: Am. Physiological Soc., 1958, p. 107.

14. COON, W. W., AND E. NAGLER. The tryptophan load as a test for pyridoxine deficiency in hospitalized patients. *Ann. N. Y. Acad. Sci.* 166: 30, 1969.

15. WACHSTEIN, M., AND A. GUDAITIS. Detection of vitamin B_6 deficiency. Utilization of an improved method for rapid determination of xanthurenic acid in urine. *Am. J. Clin. Pathol.* 22: 652, 1952.

16. NOWAK, H., AND W. F. KÖRNER. Automatic determination of xanthurenic acid. *Anal. Biochem.* 17: 154, 1966.

17. DELFORGE, J. P., AND J. FERIN. A histometric study of two estrogens: ethinyl estradiol and its 3-methyl ether derivative (mestranol); their comparative effect upon the growth of the human endometrium. *Contraception* 1: 57, 1970.

18. PRICE, J. M., R. R. BROWN AND N. YESS. Testing the functional capacity of the tryptophan-niacin pathway in man by analysis of urinary metabolites, In: *Advances in Metabolic Disorders*, edited by R. Levine and R. Luft. New York: Academic, vol. II, 1965, p. 159.

19. MICHAEL, A. F., K. N. DRUMMOND, D. DOEDEN, J. A. ANDERSON AND R. A. GOOD. Tryptophan metabolism in man. *J. Clin. Invest.* 43: 1730, 1964.

20. Rose, D. P. The influence of sex, age and breast cancer upon tryptophan metabolism. *Clin. Chem. Acta* 18: 221, 1967.
21. Lepkovsky, S., E. Roboz and A. J. Haagen-Smit. Xanthurenic acid and its role in the tryptophane metabolism of pyridoxine-deficient rats. *J. Biol. Chem.* 149: 195, 1943.
22. Greenberg, L. D., D. F. Bohr, H. McGrath and J. F. Rinehart. Xanthurenic acid excretion in the human subject on a pyridoxine-deficient diet. *Arch. Biochem.* 21: 237, 1949.
23. Spiera, H. Excretion of tryptophan metabolites in rheumatoid arthritis. *Arthritis Rheum.* 9: 318, 1966.
24. Rapoport, M. I. and W. R. Beisel. Studies of tryptophan metabolism in experimental animals and man during infectious illness. *Am. J. Clin. Nutr.* July, 1971.
25. Wachstein, M., and A. Gudaitis. Disturbance of vitamin B₆ metabolism in pregnancy. *J. Lab. Clin. Med.* 40: 550, 1952.
26. Rose, D. P., and I. P. Braidman. Oral contraceptives, depression and amino acid metabolism. *Lancet* 1: 1117, 1970.
27. Brin, M. Abnormal tryptophan metabolism in pregnancy and with the oral contraceptive pill. I. Specific effects of an oral estrogenic contraceptive steroid on the tryptophan oxygenase and two aminotransferase activities in livers of ovariectomized–adrenalectomized rats. *Am. J. Clin. Nutr.* 24: 699, 1971.
28. Mason, M., J. Ford and H. L. C. Wu. Effects of steroid and nonsteroid metabolites on enzyme conformation and pyridoxal phosphate binding. *Ann. N. Y. Acad. Sci.* 166: 170, 1969.
29. Lardy, H. A. The role of tryptophan metabolites in regulating gluconeogenesis. *Am. J. Clin. Nutr.* July, 1971.
30. Quagliariello, E., and F. Palmieri. Effects of tryptophan metabolites on enzymes of oxidative phosphorylation. *Am. J. Clin. Nutr.* July, 1971.
31. Kotake, Y., and E. Murakami. A possible diabetogenic role for tryptophan metabolites and effects of xanthurenic acid on insulin. *Am. J. Clin. Nutr.* July, 1971.
32. Allen, M. J., E. Boyland, C. E. Dukes, E. S. Horning and J. G. Watson. Cancer of the urinary bladder induced in mice with metabolites of aromatic amines and tryptophan. *Brit. J. Cancer* 11: 212, 1957.
33. Bryan, G. T. The role of urinary tryptophan metabolites in the etiology of bladder cancer. *Am. J. Clin. Nutr.* July, 1971.
34. Curzon, G., and A. R. Green. Rat liver tryptophan pyrrolase activity and brain 5-hydroxytryptamine. *Biochem. J.* 111: 15P, 1969.
35. Curzon, G. Metabolic changes in depression. *Lancet* 1: 257, 1969.
36. Borsook, H. The relation of the vitamin B₆ human requirement to the amount in the diet. *Vitamins Hormones* 22: 855, 1964.
37. Recommended Dietary Allowances (7th ed.). *Natl. Acad. Sci.–Natl. Res. Council Publ.* 1694. Washington, D. C., 1968, p. 46.
38. Recommended Intakes of Nutrients for the United Kingdom. *Dept. Health Soc. Sec. Rept.* no. 120, London, 1969, p. 21.

MAGNESIUM AND CITRATE DURING THE MENSTRUAL CYCLE: EFFECT OF AN ORAL CONTRACEPTIVE ON SERUM MAGNESIUM*

N. F. GOLDSMITH, Ph.D., N. PACE, Ph.D., J. P. BAUMBERGER, Sc.D., AND H. URY, M.A.

The contraceptive use of exogenous steroids has stimulated the investigation of steroidal effects on various organ systems, including studies of serum minerals. Serum levels of iodine,[8, 16] copper,[5, 25] and iron[3, 20] are elevated in contraceptive users; calcium,[6] magnesium,[12] phosphorus,[27] and zinc[14] are lower. Mardell and Zilva[20] observed that the pattern of serum iron variation during the menstrual cycle was not changed with oral contraceptive therapy; lowest levels of serum iron in both instances occurred at the menses. In the present study, we report that serum magnesium levels are decreased at ovulation in normal women and after 8 days of Enovid usage. In addition, cyclic variations in urinary magnesium, calcium and citrate were investigated in 2 ovulating women.

METHODS

Ten ovulating women with normal menstrual history whose ages ranged from 18–38 years served as normal subjects. The women kept basal body temperature records for 1 cycle or more, counting the first day of menstrual flow as Day 1. Ovulation as indicated by a midcycle decrease in basal temperature occurred during each natural cycle under study. A 72-hr. ovulatory interval was assumed.[22] Data were collected from 4 women using Enovid 5 mg./day, menstrual Days 5 through 24. Venous blood samples were obtained generally 2 hr. after breakfast. Three subjects were scheduled for daily samples; one of these was resampled 1 year later. Seven ovulating women and 4 Enovid users were sampled 12 times in a single cycle.

Subject 1, 24 years, was unmarried; Subject 2, 38 years, was married with 4 children. Both subjects were scheduled for daily blood samples over 30 consecutive days, comprising 2 half-cycles. Total urines were collected for three 8-hr. periods, 0700–1500, 1500–2300, 2300–0700, and were stored in polyethylene at 5° C. Urine volumes were measured to the nearest 5 ml., pH was determined using short-range Hydrion paper, and an aliquot was frozen. The 2300 and 0700 aliquots were prepared at home, frozen initially at −10° C. and removed to −20° C. Seventy-two urine specimens were collected from Subject 1 (1 sample incomplete); urinary calcium was analyzed in 37 samples randomly chosen. Eighty-seven urines were collected from Subject 2 (5 incomplete); urinary calcium was analyzed in 24 daytime samples.

Microhematocrits were determined using nonheparinized tubes. Citrate was assayed by a modification of the McArdle[21] method using heptane as an extractive. In 2 trials, citrate recoveries averaged 89 ± 8 and 100 ± 7% ($N = 6$) with a tendency to underestimate the highest concentrations.

* Supported by United States Public Health Service Research Grant RG 6003.

Serum magnesium was determined by fluorometry,[29] urinary magnesium and calcium by atomic absorption;[35] coefficients of variations were less than 2%. Citrate and magnesium-calcium analyses in urine were conducted in 2 randomized orders. Absorptiometric analyses were made on single samples; all other determinations were made in duplicate.

Computations included Pearson's correlation coefficient, Kendall's[17] coefficient of concordance applied to ranked sums and inversion test for trend, and rank sum multiple comparisons.[23] Summary data are mean ± 1 S.D.

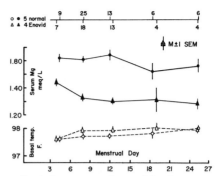

FIG. 2. Serum magnesium and basal temperature data from 5 ovulating women and 4 Enovid users, each sampled 12 times in a single cycle. *Numbers* as in Fig. 1. In ovulating women serum magnesium was lower by ~0.10 mEq./L. on Day 18 compared to Days 4 and 8. In contraceptive users, serum magnesium decreased 0.14 mEq./L. during the first 8 days of drug use.

RESULTS

Serum Magnesium in Ovulating Women and Enovid Users. Serum magnesium was analyzed in 172 blood samples taken from 10 women during 11 menstrual cycles or contiguous half-cycles. The results were summed by 3-day intervals of the cycle and distributed around menstrual Day 15, the day of lowest average basal body temperature (Fig. 1). Mean serum magnesium concentrations were lower by approximately 0.15 mEq./L. on Day 18 of the menstrual cycle compared to Days 6, 9, and 27.

Serum magnesium was significantly lower at ovulation in data from 6 women. In these women, observations of serum magnesium concentrations were made at least

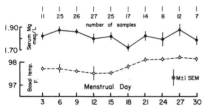

FIG. 1. Serum magnesium and basal temperature data from 10 ovulating women. Menses Days 1–5; ovulation, Day 15; cycle length, 28.5 days. *Numbers* refer to samples analyzed per group of days. Serum magnesium was ~0.15 mEq./L. lower on Day 18 compared to Days 6, 9, and 27.

once in each of 5 5-day time intervals centered about Days 5, 10, 15 (ovulation), 20, and 25. Data from 1 subject resampled after 1 year were combined; 4 women were lost because no data were available for an internal time period. Serum magnesium values for each interval were averaged and then ranked for each subject. Kendall's coefficient of concordance was applied to these ranks, giving $W = 182.5$, $p < 0.01$. A follow-up rank sum multiple comparison indicated that serum magnesium was significantly lower on Day 15 than on Day 5, or Day 25, $p < 0.03$.[23]

For comparison, the data from 5 ovulating women and 4 Enovid users, each sampled 12 times in a single cycle, were summed by 5-day intervals (Fig. 2). In the ovulating women, serum magnesium was again 0.10–0.12 mEq./L. lower on Day 18 compared to menstrual and follicular levels. Enovid users showed a decrease of 0.14 mEq./L. in serum magnesium after starting the drug (Day 3.9, 1.64 mEq./L.; Day 12.4, 1.50 mEq./L.).

Serum magnesium in the contraceptive users underwent a significant decline during Days 1–12 of the cycle. For each

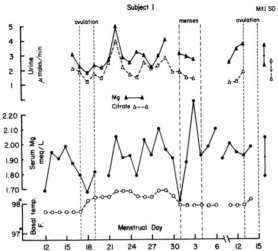

Subject 1   M±1 SD

FIG. 3. Subject 1. Average values for urinary magnesium and citrate, serum magnesium and basal temperature during 2 contiguous half cycles.

woman, 1 or 2 serum magnesium analyses were obtained during the first 5 days and 6 or 7 analyses for Days 6 through 12. These data were ranked and the ranks for all subjects on each day were summed. Serum magnesium was probably higher on Day 5, p < 0.05 (observations available for 3 out of 4 women, outlier test of Thompson and Willke[32]). According to Kendall's inversion test for trend, serum magnesium in each subject showed a tendency to decrease with time; in one woman this was significant at the 5% level. The combined rank score ratio (observed − expected result/S.D.) was 2.42, p < 0.005.

Mean basal temperatures increased 0.6° F. during the ovulation-luteal shift in ovulating women (Fig. 1) and were persistently higher in the contraceptive users during drug usage (Fig. 2).

Relation of Serum Magnesium to Urinary Magnesium, Calcium, and Citrate in 2 Subjects. Subjects 1 and 2 began the experiment on Days 12 and 13 respectively and continued to ovulation of a second cycle (Figs. 3 and 5). Twenty-nine 20-ml.

blood samples were withdrawn from each subject, approximately 15% of total blood volume. Mean hematocrit readings (Table 1) indicated fair toleration of the blood loss. However, Subject 2 showed a decrease in hematocrit with time (experiment day vs. hematocrit r = 0.388, N of 24, p < 0.05) and both subjects reported a delay of 2–3 days in the expected onset of the second cycle. Computed data are summarized in Table 1.

Figures 3 and 5 show basal temperature, serum magnesium, and mean values for urinary magnesium and citrate plotted according to menstrual day for the 2 subjects. Figures 4 and 6 show the urinary magnesium and citrate values separately for morning, evening, and night urine samples; urinary calcium is shown for the 0700–1500 interval (Fig. 6). Ovulation occurred Day 17 and Day 13 in the partial cycles of Subject 1 and Day 13 and probably Day 10 for Subject 2.

In both subjects, serum magnesium started at a low point (≤ M − 1 S.D.) during ovulation and rose irregularly to a

58

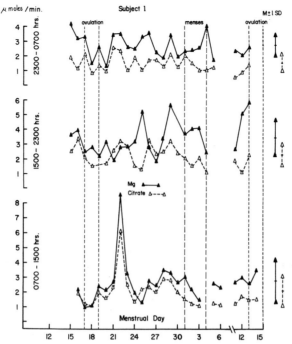

FIG. 4. Subject 1. Urinary magnesium and citrate excretion, micromoles per minute. Samples collected 0700-1500, 1500-2300 and 2300-0700 during the menstrual cycle.

high value ($\geq M$ + 1 S.D.) just before the menses and then fell. The serum magnesium peaks, Days 22 and 28 in Subject 1 and Day 28 in Subject 2, were coincident with very high or highest readings of basal temperature and peaks ($\geq M$ + 2 S.D.) of urinary magnesium and citrate excretion, concurrent or within 24 hr. It should be noted that, although the 2 subjects were studied at the same time, the peak complexes did not occur on the same calendar day. In both subjects, lowest serum magnesium values during ovulation were associated with low or lowest urinary magnesium and citrate excretion. During ovulation and the luteal half-cycles in 1 or both subjects, serum magnesium changes were related to fluctuations in urinary magnesium, citrate, calcium, pH, and basal temperature 0.05 > p > 0.001 (Table 1). Subject 1 showed a negative correlation of serum magnesium with urinary pH; urinary magnesium and citrate were highly correlated in her daytime samples (Fig. 4, 23 samples, $r = 0.896$, p ≪ 0.001).

DISCUSSION

The 28–29-day menstrual cycle can be divided into a 5-day menstruation, 8-day preovulatory or follicular phase, 6-day ovulatory period, and 10-day luteal phase.[19] The ovulatory interval thus extends on either side of the 3-day low temperature-egg extrusion that we employed in Figs. 3–6. The hormonal temperature sequence at ovulation begins with an estrogen peak, followed by the basal temperature nadir, peaks of follicle-stimulating

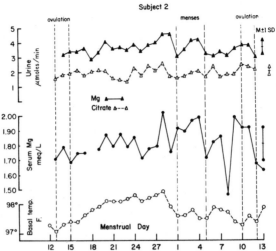

FIG. 5. Subject 2. Average values for urinary magnesium and citrate, serum magnesium and basal temperature during 2 contiguous half-cycles.

hormone, luteinizing hormone, and growth hormone, and the start of the sustained progesterone rise and temperature elevation associated with the luteal phase.[7, 10, 19, 22, 24] Our results showed that serum and urinary magnesium were lower at ovulation. In 1 subject there was an associated decrease of urinary citrate and calcium; this was accompanied by normal urine flows (not shown).

The ovulatory decreases of serum and urinary magnesium and urinary citrate may be related to the preovulatory estrogen peak. Serum magnesium and urinary citrate were lower during the middle of the menstrual cycle.[30, 34] Serum calcium showed no significant changes during the cycle,[26] but after therapeutic doses of estrogen, calcium, and phosphorus were diminished and mineral storage occurred.[1] Although a calcitonin parathyroid interaction is not excluded,[9] in mice estrogen effects on calcium retention were not mediated by the parathyroids.[13] Conceivably, serum and urinary magnesium decreases at ovulation could be related to the concurrent luteinizing hormone and follicle-stimulating hormone peaks, but a gonadotropin effect on mineral retention probably requires an active gonad.[13, 31]

More convincingly, estrogen treatment of postmenopausal osteoporotics provides almost quantitative comparison with our results: after 5 days of ethinyl estradiol 0.1–0.2 mg./day, serum calcium declined 0.15 mEq./L.[36] Ovulating women secrete endogenous estrogens at the rate of 0.2–0.5 mg. per day[2]; Enovid users in this study were being treated with 3-methyl-ethinylestradiol (mestranol) 0.075 mg./day. In ovulating women at ovulation, 1–3 days after a putative estrogen peak, and in contraceptive users after 8 days of pill ingestion, the observed decreases in serum magnesium were ~0.15 mEq./L. It seems likely therefore that reduced serum levels of magnesium at ovulation and of both magnesium and calcium after contraceptive therapy may be the results of estrogen activity.

TABLE 1. *Computed Data on 2 Women*

	Subject 1	p <*	Subject 2	p <*
Age, yr.	24.2		38.5	
Cycle lengths, days	30, 33	0.02	29, 25	
Experiment days†	23		29	
Basal temperature, ° F	98.1 ± 0.2		97.8 ± 0.3	0.02
Blood				
Sampling time, hr.	10.0 ± 0.7 (22)		9.9 ± 0.8 (28)	
Serum Mg, mEq./L.	1.91 ± 0.14 (22)		1.81 ± 0.12 (28)	
Hematocrit, %	44 ± 2 (17)		41 ± 2 (23)	
Urines				
Daily volume, ml.	1190 ± 345		1130 ± 265	
pH‡	6.1 ± 0.2	−0.005	6.0 ± 0.3	
Mg,‡ μmoles/min.	2.9 ± 0.7 (20)	0.05	3.5 ± 0.5 (28)	0.02
Citrate,‡ μmoles/min.	1.9 ± 0.6 (21)	0.01	1.9 ± 0.3 (28)	
Calcium,§ μmoles/min.	2.1 ± 1.1 (20)	0.02		
0700–1500 volume, ml.	355 ± 125		620 ± 230	
pH	6.0 ± 0.3	−0.005	6.2 ± 0.4	
Mg, μmoles/min.	2.7 ± 1.5 (22)	0.02	4.0 ± 1.1	
Citrate, μmoles/min.	2.0 ± 1.0 (22)	0.02	2.4 ± 0.6	
Calcium, μmoles/min.	2.1 ± 1.3 (11)		1.1 ± 0.4 (24)	
1500–2300 volume, ml.	515 ± 200		310 ± 0.7	
pH	6.2 ± 0.4		6.1 ± 0.4	
Mg, μmoles/min.	3.4 ± 1.2 (21)		3.6 ± 0.7	
Citrate, μmoles/min.	2.2 ± 0.7 (22)	0.02	2.1 ± 0.5	
Calcium, μmoles/min.	2.5 ± 1.3 (15)			
2300–0700 volume, ml.	315 ± 130		200 ± 70	
pH	6.0 ± 0.3		5.7 ± 0.4	
Mg, μmoles/min.	2.6 ± 0.7		2.8 ± 0.8	0.001
Citrate, μmoles/min.	1.4 ± 0.6		1.1 ± 0.3	
Calcium, μmoles/min.	1.4 ± 0.5 (9)			

* p <—Significant correlations are shown for serum magnesium during ovulation and the luteal half-cycles only; Subject 1, 15 samples; Subject 2, 17 samples. Minus sign indicates negative correlation with serum magnesium.

† Numbers of samples are shown in parentheses if not identical with experiment days.

‡ Mean of 3 values per day.

§ Mean of 1–3 values per day.

The serum minerals can thus be divided on the basis of their response to the oral contraceptives. The protein carrier-bound group, iodine, iron, and copper, are increased after contraceptive therapy probably due to estrogen-induced synthesis of the carriers and presumable release of mineral stores. The noncarrier or osseous mineral group, calcium, magnesium, phosphorus, and zinc, are decreased after contraceptive therapy, possibly due to estrogen inhibition of bone resorption.[18] An estrogen effect has been demonstrated for calcium and phosphorus[27, 36]; further studies are needed for zinc[14, 25] and magnesium. If the observed declines in serum magnesium, urinary magnesium, calcium, and citrate at ovulation represent, in fact, inhibition of bone resorption, growth hormone[13] or compensatory parathyroid secretion[9] may reinitiate the resorptive process. Alternatively, *intracellular* binding of magnesium and phosphorus may occur, possibly due to increased protein synthesis.[33]

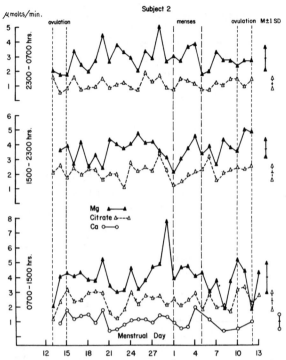

FIG. 6. Subject 2. Urinary magnesium and citrate excretion, micromoles per minute. Samples collected as described in Fig. 4. Urinary calcium excretion during 0700–1500.

Serum magnesium concentrations were positively correlated with basal temperature during ovulation and the luteal half-cycle (Table 1, Subject 2), but whether serum magnesium increases are a cause or an effect of increased heat content is difficult to decide. Serum magnesium and oral temperatures in normal subjects increased in parallel in a single day.[15] Subnormal temperatures, recorded in a case of magnesium-protein deficiency, returned to normal after magnesium therapy.[4] In normal animals, magnesium injections resulted in increased heat dissipation and inhibition of shivering,[15] and thus a decrease in heat content.

Progesterone is known to act on the central nervous system to produce the luteal increases in basal temperature[28] and, theoretically, secondary increases in serum magnesium. In the contraceptive users, norethynodrel has a thermogenic effect,[28] but the estrogen component mestranol and possibly the estrogenicity of norethynodrel may prevent magnesium release from osseous sites.[11]

SUMMARY

Serum magnesium concentrations in 10 normal women were ~0.15 mEq./L. lower during the ovulatory phase of the menstrual cycle compared to follicular or luteal phases. Nonparametric analysis of data from 6 of these women showed that the serum magnesium decrease at ovulation was significant, $p < 0.03$. In women using a combined oral contraceptive, serum magnesium decreased ∼0.15 mEq./L. during the first 8 days of drug use, p < 0.01. In 2 women the serum magnesium decline at ovulation was accompanied by decreased excretion of urinary magnesium and citrate. Serum magnesium increased during the luteal phase, accompanied by corresponding increases in basal temperature and urinary magnesium, calcium and citrate, 0.05 > p > 0.001. In 1 subject, urinary magnesium and citrate were excreted with a high degree of correlation, p ≪ 0.001. The theory is advanced that the magnesium decreases at ovulation and in the contraceptive users are the result of estrogen activity.

Acknowledgments. Dr. H. S. Winters collaborated in the studies of the contraceptive users. The absorption spectrophotometer was provided by Dr. T. Arkley.

REFERENCES

1. ALBRIGHT, F., AND REIFENSTEIN, E. C., JR. *The Parathyroid Glands and Metabolic Bone Disease.* Williams & Wilkins, Baltimore, 1948, p. 150.
2. BAIRD, D. T. A method for the measurement of estrone and estradiol-17β in peripheral human blood and other biological fluids using ³⁵S pipsyl chloride. *J Clin Endocr 28:* 244, 1968.
3. BURTON, J. L. Effect of oral contraceptives on haemoglobin, packed-cell volume, serum-iron and total iron-binding capacity in healthy women. *Lancet 1:*978, 1967.
4. CADDELL, J. L. Magnesium deficiency *in extremis. Nutr Today 2:*14, 1967.
5. CARRUTHERS, M. E., HOBBS, C. B., AND WARREN, R. L. Raised serum copper and caeruloplasmin levels in subjects taking oral contraceptives. *J Clin Path 19:*498, 1966.
6. COLLEN, M. F. Preventive Health Services Research Program, Annual Report, CD-00142-02, 1967.
7. FAIMAN, C., AND RYAN, R. J. Serum follicle-stimulating hormone and luteinizing hormone concentrations during the menstrual cycle as determined by radioimmunoassays. *J Clin Endocr 27:*1711, 1967.
8. FLORSHEIM, W. H., AND FAIRCLOTH, M. A. Effects of oral ovulation inhibitors on serum

protein-bound iodine and thyroxin binding proteins. *Proc Soc Exp Biol Med 117:*56, 1964.
9. FOSTER, G. V., JOPLIN, G. F., MACINTYRE, I., MELVIN, K. E. W., AND STACK, E. Effects of thyrocalcitonin in man. *Lancet 1:*107, 1966.
10. FRANTZ, A. G., AND RABKIN, M. T. Effects of estrogen and sex difference on secretion of human growth hormone. *J Clin Endocr 25:* 1470, 1965.
11. GOLDSMITH, N. F., AND BAUMBERGER, J. P. Mineral changes after norethynodrel. *Lancet 2:* 567, 1967.
12. GOLDSMITH, N. F., AND GOLDSMITH, J. R. Epidemiological aspects of magnesium and calcium metabolism. Implications of altered magnesium metabolism in women taking drugs for the suppression of ovulation. *Arch Environ Hlth (Chicago) 12:*607, 1966.
13. GORDAN, G. S., HANSEN, J., AND LUBICH, W. "Effects of Hormonal Steroids on Osteolysis." In *Proceedings of the 2nd International Congress on Hormonal Steroids,* Milan, 1966, p. 786.
14. HALSTEAD, J. A., HACKLEY, B. M., AND SMITH, J. C., JR. Plasma-zinc and copper in pregnancy and after oral contraceptives. *Lancet 2:*278, 1968.
15. HEAGY, F. C., AND BURTON, A. C. Effect of intravenous injection of magnesium chloride on the body temperature of the unanesthetized dog, with some observations on magnesium levels and body temperature in man. *Amer J Physiol 152:*407, 1948.
16. HOLLANDER, C. S., GARCIA, A. M., STURGIS, S. H., AND SELENKOW, H. A. Effect of an ovulatory suppressant on the serum protein-bound iodine and the red-cell uptake of radioactive tri-iodothyronine. *New Eng J Med 269:*501, 1963.
17. KENDALL, M. G. *Rank Correlation Methods.* Hafner, New York, 1962.
18. LINDQUIST, B., BUDY, A. M., MCLEAN, F. C., AND HOWARD, J. L. Skeletal metabolism in estrogen-treated rats studied by means of Ca⁴⁵. *Endocrinology 66:*100, 1960.
19. LORAINE, J. A., AND BELL, E. T. Hormone excretion during the normal menstrual cycle. *Lancet 1:*1340, 1963.
20. MARDELL, M., AND ZILVA, J. F. Effect of oral contraceptives on the variation in serum-iron during the menstrual cycle. *Lancet 2:* 1323, 1963.
21. MCARDLE, B. A modified method for the microdetermination of citric acid. *Biochem J 60:*647, 1955.

22. McArthur, J. W., Worcester, J., and Ingersoll, F. M. The urinary excretion of interstitial-cell and follicle-stimulating hormone activity during the normal menstrual cycle. *J Clin Endocr 18:*1186, 1958.
23. McDonald, B. J., and Thompson, W. A., Jr. Rank sum multiple comparisons in one- and two-way classifications. *Biometrika 54:* 487, 1967.
24. Neill, J. D., Johannson, E. D. B., Datta, J. K., and Knobil, E. Relationship between the plasma levels of luteinizing hormone and progesterone during the normal menstrual cycle. *J Clin Endocr 27:*1167, 1967.
25. O'Leary, J. A., and Spellacy, W. N. Zinc and copper levels in pregnant women and those taking oral contraceptives. *Amer J Obstet Gynec 103:*131, 1969.
26. Philips, R. S., McCoord, A. B., and Pommerenke, W. T. Serum electrolytes in the menstrual cycle. *Fertil Steril 3:*402, 1952.
27. Pulkkinen, M. O., and Willman, K. Oral contraceptives and phosphorus metabolism. *Brit Med J 2:*574, 1967.
28. Rothchild, I. Interrelations between progesterone and the ovary, pituitary and central nervous system in the control of ovulation and the regulation of progesterone secretion. *Vitamins Hormones 23:*248, 1965.
29. Schachter, D. Fluorometric estimation of magnesium with 8-hydroxy-5-quinolinesulfonate. *J Lab Clin Med 58:*495, 1961.
30. Shorr, E., Bernheim, A. R., and Taussky, H. The relation of urinary citric acid excretion to the menstrual cycle and the steroidal reproductive hormones. *Science 95:*606, 1942.
31. Smith, R. W., Jr. Dietary and hormonal factors in bone loss. *Fed Proc 26:*1737, 1967.
32. Thompson, W. A., Jr., and Willke, T. A. On an extreme rank sum test for outliers. *Biometrika 50:*375, 1963.
33. Ui, H. and Mueller, G. C. The role of RNA synthesis in the mechanism of estrogen action. *Fed Proc 22:*409, 1963.
34. von Nida, S., and Broja, E. Die hormonale Beeinflussung des Magnesium- und Calcium-blutspiegels während des Menstruationscyclus. *Arch Gynäk 188:*247, 1957.
35. Willis, J. B. Analysis of biological materials by atomic absorption spectroscopy (In D. Glick, ed.). *Meth Biochem Anal 11:*1, 1963.
36. Young, M. M., Jasani, C., Smith, D. A., and Nordin, B. E. C. Some effects of ethinyl oestradiol on calcium and phosphorus metabolism in osteoporosis. *Clin Sci 34:*411, 1968.

64

THE EFFECT OF AN ORAL CONTRACEPTIVE AGENT
ON THE CONCENTRATIONS OF CALCIUM AND MAGNESIUM
IN PLASMA, ERYTHROCYTES AND PLATELETS IN WOMEN

C. G. THIN

INTRODUCTION

Thrombosis associated with magnesium depletion has been described by Allanby et al. (1) and Durlach (4,5). Durlach reported a particularly striking loss of calcium and magnesium from blood platelets and drew attention to the suggestion that pregnancy and anti-ovulatory drugs (7) lower the concentration of magnesium in serum.

As it has been shown that thrombotic disease is a risk attending the use of oral contraceptives (6), it was decided to study the effects of such an agent on calcium and magnesium concentrations in the components of blood of a group of women using a drug of this type.

Evidence regarding the normal levels of calcium and magnesium to be found in blood platelets is limited. In addition, therefore, to the treated group we also determined the mean value and range in a group of normal untreated women. The effect of the normal menstrual cycle on the levels of calcium and magnesium in blood was also studied for purposes of comparison with treated group.

PATIENTS AND METHODS

Blood was obtained from 41 normal untreated volunteers in order to provide a range of normal values. To study the effect of the menstrual cycle blood was taken from 19 females aged 17—42 years on day 5 and day 20 of the cycle. None of the females in either group was taking an oral contraceptive.

'Gynovlar' was the anti-ovulatory drug chosen for study because it has been widely used for several years, and because it contains an oestro-

65

TABLE 1

Estimates of precision of the methods used expressed as the estimates of (s) of results of duplicate determinations.

	Number of duplicates	Range covered	s
Magnesium in red blood cell mg/g cells	41	3.61—5.61	0.12
Calcium in platelets mg/g dry wt	38	1.03—3.63	0.23
Magnesium in platelets mg/g dry wt	38	0.32—0.77	0.05

$$s^2 = \pm \frac{(\text{difference between duplicate determinations})^2}{2 \times \text{number of duplicates}}$$

gen, though in small amounts, ethinyl oestradiol 0.05 mg with norethisterone acetate 3 mg.

Volunteers for the study with 'Gynovlar' were obtained through the Family Planning Centre. Blood samples were taken immediately before initiating treatment, and at intervals of 3 months, 6 months and 1 year thereafter. Blood was taken on the penultimate day of the appropriate course of treatment. In order to provide effective comparisons with the treated group an additional group of volunteers was also studied. This group was matched for age and parity with the treated group but had been on treatment with 'Gynovlar' for 1—4 years.

Separation of red blood cells and platelets

50 ml of blood was taken from the antecubital vein into disposable plastic syringes and was then carefully transferred to two 25 ml siliconised glass bottles containing 0.2 ml heparin. These were centrifuged immediately at room temperature for 15 minutes at 700—900 rpm in a swing-out head. The top 2/3 of the platelet-rich plasma obtained in this way was removed from each bottle with a siliconised pipette and transferred to 5 ml plastic centrifuge tubes for further separation of the platelets.

The red blood cell layer was centrifuged further and washed three times with physiological saline, the final centrifugation being at 2,800 rpm for 1 hour. Weighed aliquots of the packed cells, about 1 g, were diluted to 25 ml with glass distilled water and the magnesium content determined by atomic absorption spectrophotometry (8).

The platelet-rich supernatant plasma was centrifuged at 750 g for 20 minutes at 4 C and the platelets were washed and recentrifuged three times with physiological saline. After the final centrifugation the tubes were drained, and the platelets transferred with 97 % alcohol to small tared platinum crucibles. After drying overnight in an oven at 100—110 C the dry weight of the platelets was determined, they were then ashed at 500 C for 12 hours. The ash was taken up in 0.6—1.0 ml 0.1 N HCl, the volume used depending on the weight of platelets obtained. The calcium and magnesium content was determined by atomic absorption spectrophotometry (8).

Plasma calcium and magnesium were also determined by atomic absorption spectrophotometry (8). The plasma calcium concentration was corrected where necessary to a specific gravity of 1.027(3).

RESULTS

The precision of the methods used is shown in Table 1 and the mean and calculated range of normal values in Table 2. The values found are not identical with, but are similar to, those reported by Cousin and Caen (2).

The effect of the menstrual cycle on the parameters studied is shown in Table 3. No significant differences were found between results obtained on day 5 of the cycle and those obtained on day 20.

Among twenty volunteers studied, 10 (Group A) continued on treatment for at least 6 months, and of these 10, only 5 continued for 1 year. Ten other volunteers (Group B) who had been on treatment with Gynovlar for 1—4 years were matched for age and parity with Group A. The age range in both groups was 19—38 years. Though the numbers are small, an analysis of variance was carried out and no significant differences in any of the parameters studied was found. The results are shown in Table 4.

DISCUSSION

Alterations in the concentrations of naturally occurring hormones, as occurs in the menstrual cycle, does not appear to affect the levels of calcium or magnesium

66

TABLE 2

The distribution, actual range and calculated range (within 95 % confidence limits) of normal values of calcium and magnesium in blood constituents.

	Number of samples	Actual range	Mean ± SD	Calculated range P < 0.05
Serum calcium[1] mg/100 ml	137	8.15—10.25	9.23 ± 0.43	8.38—10.08
Serum magnesium[1] mg/100 ml	138	1.70— 2.65	2.13 ± 0.15	1.83— 2.43
Red blood cell magnesium mg/g cells	41	3.61— 5.61	4.47 ± 0.41	3.65— 5.29
Platelet calcium mg/g dry wt	38	1.03— 3.63	1.98 ± 0.48	1.02— 2.94
Platelet magnesium mg/g dry wt	38	0.32— 0.77	0.50 ± 0.074	0.35— 0.65
Platelet calcium[2] mg/g dry wt	15	1.23— 3.90	2.92 ± 0.95	1.02— 4.72
Platelet magnesium[2] mg/g dry wt	20	0.20— 0.39	0.3 ± 0.065	0.17— 0.43

[1] Thin and Thomson (8). Plasma used throughout this experiment.
[2] Cousin and Caen (2).

TABLE 3

The effect of the oestrous cycle on calcium and magnesium levels in blood constituents.

	Day of cycle	Number of subjects	Mean	Variance	t	Significance
Plasma calcium mg/100 ml	5	18	9.46	0.1505	0.17	n.s.
	20	18	9.44	0.0975		
Plasma magnesium mg/100 ml	5	18	1.91	0.0071	0.41	n.s.
	20	18	1.90	0.0058		
Red blood cell magnesium mg/g	5	19	4.38	0.1693	0.01	n.s.
	20	19	4.37	0.0879		
Platelet calcium mg/g dry wt	5	17	2.17	0.2148	0.13	n.s.
	20	17	2.00	0.1585		
Platelet magnesium mg/g dry wt	5	17	0.53	0.0053	0.14	n.s.
	20	17	0.50	0.0055		

TABLE 4

The effect of treatment with 'Gynovlar' on calcium and magnesium in blood constituents (mean levels).

	GROUP A				GROUP B After treatment for 1—4 years
	Pre-treatment	After treatment for			
		3 months	6 months	1 year	
Number of subjects	10	10	10	5	10
Plasma calcium mg/100 ml	9.47	9.34	9.46	9.60	9.61
Plasma magnesium mg/100 ml	1.98	1.98	1.92	1.95	1.93
Red blood cell magnesium mg/g cells	4.42	4.09	4.41	4.60	4.63
Platelet calcium mg/g dry wt	1.24	1.63	1.60	1.49	1.94
Platelet magnesium mg/g dry wt	0.34	0.47	0.47	0.43	0.47
Platelets/100 ml whole blood	214,000	250,000	195,000	250,000	186,000

in plasma or other constituents of whole blood. Treatment with an oral contraceptive agent, 'Gynovlar', for periods of 1—4 years does not appear to have any detectable effect on calcium or magnesium, in blood constituents either. When the level of platelet magnesium was high in the pre-treatment sample it remained high, when low it remained low, throughout treatment.

Lowenstein (7) reported that treatment with the oral contraceptive agent 'Enovid' lowered serum magnesium levels. This agent contains 10 mg norethynodrel and 0.15 mg ethinyl oestradiol — 3 methyl ether in each dose compared with 0.05 mg ethinyl oestradiol and 3 mg norethisterone acetate in each dose of 'Gynovlar'. It is possible that with the higher dose of oestrogen treatment these drugs could affect calcium and magnesium levels in the constituents of blood, while a lower dose might fail to elicit a response.

The effects of treatment with 'Gynovlar' for periods of 1 to 4 years on the levels of calcium in plasma and platelets, and magnesium in plasma, platelets and red-blood cells appears to be so small as not to be detectable in this survey.

None of the subjects studied had a thrombosis, it is possible that the levels of calcium and magnesium in women predisposed to have a thrombosis are affected by the drug.

ACKNOWLEDGEMENTS

The author wishes to thank Professor J. A. Strong for his constant encouragement, and the staff of the Edinburgh Family Planning Centre, in particular Dr. Loudon and Mrs. Macdonald, for their generous help. The author is grateful to Miss V. Smith for her excellent technical help.

REFERENCES

1. *Allanby KD, Huntsman RG, Sacker LS:* Thrombotic microangiopathy. Recovery of a case after heparin and magnesium therapy. Lancet 1: 237, 1966
2. *Cousin C, Caen J:* Dosage au magnesium et du calcium dans les plaquettes sanguines humaines. Rev Franc Etud Clin Biol 9: 520, 1964
3. *Dent CE:* Some problems of hyperparathyroidism. Brit Med J 2: 1419, 1962
4. *Durlach JA:* Le role anti thrombosique physiologique du magnesium. Coeur Med Intern 6: 213, 1967
5. *Durlach JA:* Magnesium deficiency thrombosis. Lancet 1: 1382, 1967
6. *Inman WHW, Vessey MP, Westerholm B, Engelund A:* Thromboembolic disease and the steroidal content of oral contraceptives. A report to the committee on safety of drugs. Brit Med J 2: 203, 1970
7. *Lowenstein E:* Oral contraceptives and cardiovascular disease. Lancet 2: 1365, 1966
8. *Thin CG, Thomson PA:* Estimation of calcium and magnesium in serum and urine by atomic absorption spectrophotometry. J Clin Path 20: 280, 1967

Effect of varying dosages of ethynodiol diacetate upon serum luteinizing hormone

DANIEL R. MISHELL, JR., M.D.

WILLIAM D. ODELL, M.D., PH.D.

OVULATION IN WOMEN is preceded by a mid-cycle surge of LH. It is generally believed that this surge is required for and initiates ovulation. It has been shown with the use of both bioassays and immunoassays that the combination estrogen-progestogen oral contraceptive drugs inhibit this ovulatory mid-cycle surge of luteinizing hormone (LH).[1-4] In earlier studies from our laboratories, consistent inhibition of peak levels of LH was not observed when a sequential type of oral contraceptive was administered (estrogen alone followed by estrogen plus progestogen),[5, 6] and it has been suggested that estrogen treatment may actually stimulate LH release.[5, 7]

In contrast to these findings, it has been shown that when progestogens are administered without estrogen they can inhibit the ovulatory LH peak, provided that a sufficient dosage of the progestogen is utilized. Taymor[8] found that 2.5 and 5 mg. of norethisterone acetate administered orally from Day 5 to 25 caused obliteration of the high mid-cycle levels of urinary LH excretion. Furthermore, in other studies from our laboratories[9, 10] it has been shown that 150 mg. of medroxyprogesterone acetate administered in a long-acting form intramuscularly causes inhibition of the ovulatory LH peak for periods of more than 120 days. In contrast to these observations, Elstein[11] reported that when a lower dosage of progestogen was utilized, the mid-cycle LH peak was not always inhibited. In 7 of 9 cycles during which 4 women received 0.5 mg. of chlormadinone acetate daily, a mid-cycle LH peak occurred; in each of these 7 cycles there was presumptive evidence that ovulation had occurred.

It is the purpose of this report to demonstrate the effect of various dosages of ethynodiol diacetate, a potent, orally effective progestogen, upon serum LH concentrations.

Supported by National Institutes of Health Grant HD 02701 and grants from the Ford Foundation and the G. D. Searle Company.

Materials and methods

Ethynodiol diacetate. Ethynodiol diacetate, a 17α-ethynyl-4-estrene-3β, 17β-diol diacetate, is the 3, 17 diacetate of the reduced form of norethindrone. This compound is a potent progestogen as determined by the Clauberg assay. Buccal administration of this compound in rabbits revealed it to be about 40 times more potent than progesterone.[12] In humans, Greenblatt and Mahesh[13] have shown this compound to have at least twice the progestational activity of norethindrone. Ethynodiol diacetate has only a slight estrogenic effect. It was found that this compound when administered subcutaneously has approximately 4 per cent of the estrogenic potency of estrone as determined by 2 assays. One of these assays is based on the increase of uterine weight in immature mice and the other is based on the induction of vaginal cornification in ovariectomized mature rats.[12] Ethynodiol diacetate has only very minimal androgenic activity; treatment of castrated male rats produced increases in weight of the ventral prostate only with the highest doses utilized, 2 to 20 mg. per rat. The increase in ventral prostate weights obtained with these doses was only slightly greater than that obtained with equal doses of progesterone. When compared with testosterone propionate in the same assay, it was found that the androgenicity of this compound does not exceed one per cent of testosterone propionate.[14]

Subject selection. A group of 8 women between the ages of 20 and 35 who had regular cyclic menses was selected for study. Prior to receiving medication, it had been determined that 4 of these subjects had ovulated, as judged by changes in basal body temperature, urinary pregnanediol, and endometrial biopsy. In addition, during pretreatment cycles, each of these 4 subjects demonstrated a typical mid-cycle rise in LH as determined by radioimmunoassay on serum samples obtained daily (Fig. 1). The remaining 4 subjects all had biphasic basal temperature curves in the cycle preceding treatment, but daily LH samples were not obtained. Beginning on the fifth day after

the onset of menses, tablets of ethynodiol diacetate were administered daily for 21 days to each of these 8 subjects. Following a 7 day interval without medication, each subject received the same dosage of drug for an additional 21 days. Following a 2 month interval for recovery from the effects of this dosage of drug, 7 of the 8 subjects received a different dosage for an additional 2 month period, again beginning on the fifth day of menstruation. One additional subject (D. S.) was enrolled for this 2 month period to replace the subject who left the study (P. K.). The new subject also had a history of cyclic menses and a biphasic temperature curve in the pretreatment cycle. The drug was again administered daily for 21 day periods with a 7 day interval. In the interval between medication cycles, all subjects had biphasic temperature curves. During each 2 month period in which the drug was being administered, serum samples were obtained daily and assayed for LH by a previously described radioimmunoassay method.[15, 16] The total volume of serum in all tubes in the assay was kept constant by adding dog serum to those tubes containing less serum than others. All samples from each 2 month study period were assayed together. The intraassay and interassay coefficients of variation were 2.5 and 18 per cent, respectively. The dosage of drug for the 16 two-month

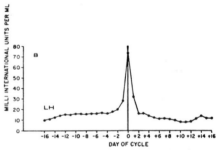

Fig. 1. Mean LH concentrations measured daily in 10 women throughout the menstrual cycle. Redrawn from Odell, Ross, and Rayford.[16] All data are centered about the mid-cycle LH peak. Onset of menses occurred variably on Days −12 to −16 and +12 to +16.

Table I. Dosage of drug given to each patient per cycle

Subject	Dosage of drug per cycle (mg.)					
	1	2	3	4	5	6
D. S.	0	0	0	0	0.1	0.1
Su. C.	0.2	0.2	0	0	1.0	1.0
M. L.	0.2	0.2	0	0	1.0	1.0
Sh. C.	0.4	0.4	0	0	2.0	2.0
A. W.	0.4	0.4	0	0	2.0	2.0
D. G.	0.6	0.6	0	0	2.0	2.0
P. K.	0.6	0.6	0	0	0	0
J. D.	0.8	0.8	0	0	1.0	1.0
M. M.	0.8	0.8	0	0	0.1	0.1

periods studied was distributed according to the schedule shown in Table I.

Results

Ethynodiol diacetate at doses of 2 mg. appears to suppress LH concentrations to low values (Fig. 2). Only one value of the 165 determined on this dose of treatment exceeded 32 mIU per milliliter* (D. G. on Day 2 of treatment). The majority of the determinations were less than 10 mIU per milliliter. At doses of 1 mg. per day, 2 of 3 patients showed suppression of LH concentrations similar to that observed at the 2 mg. dosage. One had very high and variable LH concentrations, producing the bizarre pattern shown in Fig. 3 (J. D.). During each month of therapy in this subject there were at least 2 distinct surges of LH with levels greater than or equal to 60 mIU per milliliter. Both subjects who received 0.8 mg. of the drug had LH levels between 30 and 40 mIU per milliliter soon after starting the first drug course (Fig. 4). No definite surge of LH was observed on this dosage during the first drug course, and after 12 days therapy levels of LH were depressed to less than 12 mIU per milliliter. However, during the interval between drug courses, concentrations of LH rose to the 40 to 50 mIU per milliliter range. On the first day of the second course of drug,

*Milli-International Units (mIU) of the Second International Reference Preparation of Human Menopausal Gonadotropin. The potency of the National Institutes of Health study section pituitary reference preparation (LER-907) by this radioimmunuoassay was 219 IU per milligram (95 per cent limits = 186 to 252).

one subject had an LH concentration of 50 mIU per milliliter, while the other had a surge of greater than 165 mIU per milliliter of LH on the eighth day of the drug.

Both of the subjects receiving 0.6 mg. of the drug had LH concentrations between 40 and 65 mIU per milliliter during the first two days of treatment (Fig. 5). D. G. had concentrations of 20 to 35 mIU per milliliter throughout the remainder of the first treatment cycle. P. K. had a single mid-cycle surge to 75 mIU per milliliter, and then concentrations fell to less than 15 mIU per milliliter. During the second treatment cycle, all values in both subjects were less than 30 mIU per milliliter.

One of the subjects (Sh. C.) had persistently low levels of LH during treatment with 0.4 mg. of drug as well as during the 7 day treatment-free interval (Fig. 6). Most values were between 10 and 20 mIU per milliliter. This pattern is similar to that observed in the same subject when she received 2 mg. of drug. The other subject (A. W.) who received 0.4 mg. of the drug had 2 surges of LH during the first cycle of treatment, one of 130 mIU per milliliter during the sixth drug day (eleventh cycle day) and the other 5 days later. Another surge of LH was observed during the second day of drug in the second cycle. Most of the other values were between 15 and 35 mIU per milliliter. This pattern differed from the consistently low levels of LH seen when 2.0 mg. of drug was administered to this same subject. Similarly, one of the subjects who received 0.2

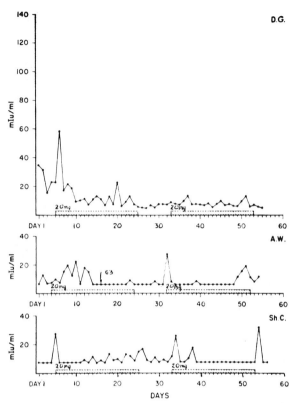

Fig. 2. Serum LH levels expressed in milli-International Units per milliliter *(mIU/ml)* of the Second International Reference Preparation of Human Menopausal Gonadotropin in 3 subjects receiving 2.0 mg. of ethynodiol diacetate for two 21 day periods (hatched horizontal bars) separated by a 7 day treatment-free interval.

mg. of drug (Su. C.) had persistently low concentrations of LH (less than 30 mIU per milliliter) similar to the pattern observed when she received 1 mg. of drug (Fig. 7). The other subject (M. L.) had a surge of LH to 75 mIU per milliliter on the seventh day of treatment during the first cycle and on the fifth day of treatment during the second cycle. This pattern differed from the suppression observed when she received 1.0 mg. of drug.

One of the subjects who received 0.1 mg. of drug had a low mid-cycle peak in the first cycle (42 mIU per milliliter) and none in the second (Fig. 8). The other patient

had a bizarre pattern of LH during therapy with numerous high peaks of LH during both courses of drug as well as in the predrug interval.

Comment

Although the number of subjects in this study was small, certain differences in the pattern of LH response to the various dosages of this progestational agent could be observed. The highest dosages of drug, 1 and 2 mg., generally caused suppression of the mid-cycle surge of high levels of LH. These findings are similar to those previously reported by Stevens and associates[2] using bio-

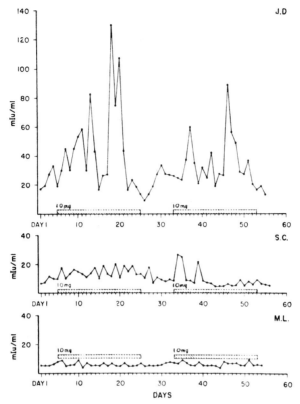

Fig. 3. Serum LH levels in 3 subjects receiving 1.0 mg. of ethynodiol diacetate for two 21 day periods (hatched horizontal bars) separated by a 7 day treatment-free interval.

assay techniques. In one subject, a single high level of LH was noted one day after she first received 2 mg. of ethynodiol diacetate. LH concentrations of subjects receiving less than 1 mg. of this drug showed a variable response that could not be related to the dose in this small number of subjects. Patterns demonstrating a mid-cycle surge of LH in either the first or second or both cycles of therapy as well as complete suppression of the LH peak were noted with these lower dosages. In addition, a surge of LH within the first few days of starting the progestogen, similar to that seen with the 2 mg. dosage, was observed several times with the lower dosage in both the initial cycle as well

as the cycle following the 7 day interval. Odell and Swerdloff[7] have demonstrated that progestogens may stimulate a surge of LH when administered to estrogen-suppressed, castrated, or postmenopausal women. This stimulation was always observed within 12 to 24 hours of the onset of progestogen treatment. In the studies reported herein in normal women, the progestogen may also have stimulated LH release. If so, it required at least 0.4 mg. of the progestogen to stimulate the LH surge within 2 days, although only 4 subjects were studied with dosages less than 0.4 mg. These findings appear to indicate that a threshold dose of this progestogen, greater than 0.4 mg. per day, is required for

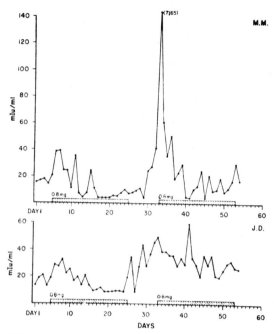

Fig. 4. Serum LH levels in 2 subjects receiving 0.8 mg. of ethynodiol diacetate for two 21 day periods (hatched horizontal bars) separated by a 7 day treatment-free interval.

stimulation of release of LH. Stevens and associates[2] reported a similar high level of LH immediately after giving one patient 0.5 mg. of this same progestational agent.

Low-dose progestogen (without estrogen) treatment has been shown to be an effective means of preventing fertility. Martinez-Manautou[17] reported results of 1,769 women who were treated with 0.5 mg. of chlormadinone acetate daily for a total of 28,158 cycles. The pregnancy rate in this study was only one per 100 woman years of use. The incidence of ovulation in patients using this method of contraception was estimated by culdoscopic observation and biopsy of ovaries[17] as well as analysis of basal temperature graphs.[18] Results of each of these studies indicated that approximately half of patients receiving 0.5 mg. of chlormadinone acetate daily had ovulatory menstrual cycles. Ovulation may also have occurred in many of the subjects

we studied. Although the drug was administered intermittently, when less than 0.5 mg. per day was given, five of the 12 cycles studied had mid-cycle peak excretions of LH which were also associated with a biphasic temperature graph. It was noted in the other 7 cycles during which low dosages of this progestogen were administered that the LH peaks were suppressed entirely or occurred at times other than mid-cycle. When the LH peak was suppressed, there was a low, flat basal temperature curve. Only one subject (during a single study cycle) who failed to have an LH peak had a biphasic temperature graph.

Although other mechanisms might be involved, this study has confirmed other studies which showed that high-dose oral progestogen treatment results in suppression of the mid-cycle LH peak. Low-dose progestogen treatment produced variable effects on serum

74

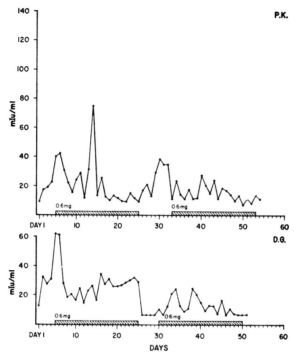

Fig. 5. Serum LH levels in 2 subjects receiving 0.6 mg. of ethynodiol diacetate for two 21 day periods (hatched horizontal bars) separated by a 7 day treatment-free interval.

LH concentrations. Some women showed LH patterns similar to those observed during the normal menstrual cycle; others showed suppression of the LH peak and failed to ovulate. Perhaps studies with large numbers of women would enable a dose-response curve to be obtained for each progestational agent used for contraceptive purposes. Correlations might be developed with parameters such as surface area or body weight so that a dosage that fails to inhibit ovulation but does inhibit fertilization could be determined for each individual women. If this were done, a daily dosage could be prescribed for each individual patient which would permit ovulation and regular menstruation, but capacity to conceive would be inhibited. Since patients receiving continuous low-dose progestational agents who fail to ovulate also

have a high incidence of prolonged cycles and probably have an increased incidence of breakthrough bleeding, such determinations would seem worthwhile.

The sequence of hormonal events occurring during the normal menstrual cycle is presently being clarified. Present knowledge has recently been summarized by Odell and Moyer,[19] Ross and colleagues,[20] and by Odell and co-workers.[21] During the first few days of the cycle, a rise in serum follicle-stimulating hormone (FSH) is observed, which presumably initiates follicle growth. During this phase as well as the remainder of the follicular phase, LH concentrations are low but rise slightly during the second half of the follicular phase. FSH falls after the initial rise to remain constant until it again rises, usually coincident with the LH peak to pro-

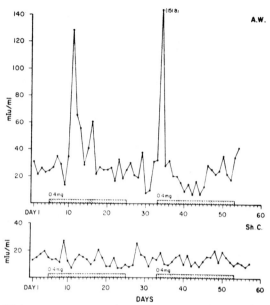

Fig. 6. Serum LH levels in 2 subjects receiving 0.4 mg. of ethynodiol diacetate for two 21 day periods (hatched horizontal bars) separated by a 7 day treatment-free interval.

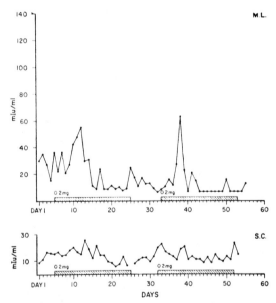

Fig. 7. Serum LH levels in 2 subjects receiving 0.2 mg. of ethynodiol diacetate for two 21 day periods (hatched horizontal bars) separated by a 7 day treatment-free interval.

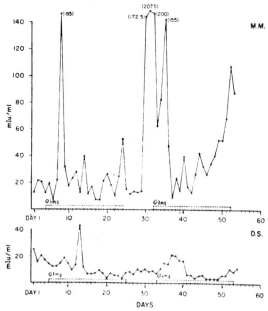

Fig. 8. Serum LH levels in 2 subjects receiving 0.1 mg. of ethynodiol diacetate for two 21 day periods (hatched horizontal bars) separated by a 7 day treatment-free interval.

duce the LH-FSH ovulation surge. After this surge, both LH and FSH fall to low and constant concentrations during the luteal phase until the corpus luteum function regresses. FSH rises during the last day or two of the cycle. These events are summarized in Fig. 1. From ovarian production, estradiol levels rise slowly and peak prior to the LH-FSH peak. Data on progesterone are conflicting; it either rises slightly before the LH-FSH peak or is very low until after the LH-FSH surge when it rapidly rises to high concentrations which persist during the luteal phase. Prevention of fertility in women might occur by interference with many aspects of this system. Odell and Moyer[19] have summarized these possibilities. For purposes of this discussion, they include, for example, abolition of the early follicular phase FSH rise and abolition of the FSH and/or the LH portions of the ovulatory peak. Inhibition of the early follicular FSH rise might lead to failure of follicle development. Thus, any

ovulatory peak that did occur might not result in ova release, since normal maturation had not occurred. In the study reported herein, it may not, therefore, be entirely accurate to call the LH surges ovulatory surges. In a small number of the patients described herein, FSH concentrations were measured; Swerdloff, Mishell, and Odell[22] found that FSH concentrations were usually suppressed during therapy.

In summary, the mechanism of this progestogen action to prevent fertility may be complex and stems from several actions. These possibly include: (1) suppression of the LH ovulatory surge, (2) stimulation of the LH surge at abnormal times, (3) suppression of either the early ovulatory rise or the mid-cycle rise in FSH or both, (4) alteration of the environment of the female reproductive tract to inhibit sperm entry or to alter ova transport, conception, migration, or implantation. Further studies are necessary to clarify these points.

REFERENCES

1. Brown, P. S., Wells, M., and Cunningham, F. J.: Lancet 2: 446, 1964.
2. Stevens, V. C., Vorys, N., Besch, P. K., and Barry, R. D.: Metabolism 14: 327, 1965.
3. Ross, G. T., Odell, W. D., and Rayford, P. L.: Lancet 2: 1255, 1966.
4. Cargille, C. M., Ross, G. T., Howland, L. A., and Rayford, P. L.: Clin. Res. 16: 33, 1968.
5. Swerdloff, R. S., and Odell, W. D.: J. Clin. Endocr. 29: 157, 1969.
6. Mishell, D. R., Jr., Talas, M., and Parlow, A. F.: Proc. 6th Annual Meeting, American Association of Planned Parenthood Physicians, Excerpta Medica International Congress Series, No. 177, 1968, p. 103.
7. Odell, W. D., and Swerdloff, R. S.: Proc. Nat. Acad. Sci. 61: 529, 1968.
8. Taymor, M. L.: J. Clin. Endocr. 24: 803, 1964.
9. Mishell, D. R., Jr.: AMER. J. OBSTET. GYNEC. 99: 86, 1967.
10. Mishell, D. R., Jr., Talas, M., Parlow, A. F., El-Habashy, M., and Moyer, D. L.: Proc. 6th World Congress of Fertility and Sterility, Israel Academy of Sciences and Humanities, Jerusalem, Israel, 1968, p. 203.
11. Elstein, M.: Proc. symp. Gonville and Caius College, Cambridge, England, Sept. 14, 1968; Syntex Pharmaceuticals, Ltd., Excerpta Medica Foundation, p. 46.
12. Elton, R. L., and Nutting, E. F.: Proc. Soc. Exp. Biol. Med. 107: 991 1961.
13. Greenblatt, R. B., and Mahesh, V. D.: Metabolism 14: 320, 1965.
14. Saunders, F. J., Nutting, E. F., Mares, S. E., and Bergstrom, R.: S. C. Ethynodiol Diacetate; A Low Progestogen: Biol. Studies, G. D. Searle and Co., 1969, p. 6.
15. Odell, W. D., Ross, G. T., and Rayford, P. L.: Metabolism 15: 287, 1966.
16. Odell, W. D., Ross, G. T., and Rayford, P. L.: J. Clin. Invest. 46: 248, 1967.
17. Martinez-Manautou, J.: Proc. symp. Gonville and Caius College, Cambridge, England, Sept. 14, 1968, Syntex Pharmaceuticals, Ltd., Excerpta Medica Foundation, p. 18.
18. MacDonald, R. R.: Proc. symp. Gonville and Caius College, Cambridge, England, Sept. 14, 1968, Syntex Pharmaceuticals, Ltd., Excerpta Medica Foundation, p. 33.
19. Odell, W. D., and Moyer, D. L.: Reproductive Physiology, St. Louis, The C. V. Mosby Company. In press.
20. Ross, G. T., Cargille, C. M., Lipsett, M. B., Rayford, P. L., Marshall, J. R., Strott, C. A., and Rodbard, D.: Recent Progr. Hormone Res. In press.
21. Odell, W. D., Swerdloff, R. S., Abraham, G. E., Jacobs, H. S., and Walsh, P. C.: Proc. 6th International Pfizer Symp., Edinburgh, Scotland, May 13-15, 1970. Edinburgh University Press. In press.
22. Swerdloff, R. S., Mishell, D. R., Jr., and Odell, W. D.: Clin. Res. 17: 110, 1969.

EFFECT OF DAILY ADMINISTRATION OF 0.5 MG. OF CHLORMADINONE ACETATE ON PLASMA LEVELS OF FOLLICLE-STIMULATING HORMONE, LUTEINIZING HORMONE, AND PROGESTERONE DURING THE MENSTRUAL CYCLE*

DOUGLAS M. SAUNDERS, M.D., STEWART L. MARCUS, M.D., BRIJ B. SAXENA, Ph.D., CARL G. BELING, M.D., AND ELIZABETH B. CONNELL, M.D.

The successful application of chlormadinone [supplied by Syntex Laboratories Inc., Palo Alto, Calif. (6-chloro-17α-hydroxypregna-4,6-diene-3,20-dione-17-acetate)], administered continuously in low dosage, has brought increasing interest in this form of contraception.[1-3] Even though the mechanism of action of chlormadinone is incompletely understood at the present time, it seems to be generally agreed upon that it does not consistently suppress ovulation.[4-7] This observation suggests the possibility that chlormadinone may exert its contraceptive action by influencing other functions such as capacitation of spermatozoa, fertilization of the ovum, or implantation of the fertilized ovum.

The aim of the present investigation was to study the changes in the plasma levels of follicle-stimulating hormone (FSH), luteinizing hormone (LH), and progesterone induced by the continuous administration of chlormadinone. Serial patterns of these hormones were used as presumptive evidence for ovulation.

MATERIALS AND METHODS

Nine healthy women were selected for this study. They all gave histories of 24–28 day regular menstrual cycles and had not been taking oral contraceptives for at least 12 months. In each woman 2 consecutive cycles were studied, the 1st cycle being the control cycle. Chlormadinone, 0.5 mg. daily, was commenced on the 1st day of the 2nd cycle and was continued for 28 days, or until the occurrence of spontaneous menstruation if delayed after the 28th day. All the subjects studied recorded basal body temperature (BBT) each morning during the control and drug trial periods. Blood was obtained daily for assessment of plasma gonadotropin and progesterone levels. In view of the large numbers of samples obtained, plasma gonadotropin levels were only determined every 2–3 days in the first and last week of the cycle, particularly where the amount of plasma was limited on that day and was required by the assay in duplicate for plasma progesterone. In order to avoid diurnal rhythmicity, blood was drawn between 9 and 9:30

* Supported by Grant 67-455 from The Ford Foundation, Grant M70.13.C from The Population Council, Grant RF-67032 from The Rockefeller Foundation, and a grant from The Josiah Macy Foundation. Presented in part at the 26th Annual Meeting of the American Fertility Society, Washington, D.C., March 18–21, 1970.

A.M. All blood samples were heparinized and centrifuged at 1500 r.p.m. for 10 min. The plasma was decanted and stored at −20° C. until assayed.

Plasma levels of FSH and LH were determined by a radioimmunoassay procedure previously described by Saxena et al.[8, 9] Highly purified human pituitary preparation, FSH[10] containing an average of 5677 I.U. of FSH/mg. and 30 I.U. of LH/mg., and LH[8] containing 5220 I.U. of LH/mg. and virtually free of FSH activity, were used as tracers and standards in the assay procedure. A pituitary FSH fraction containing 800 I.U./mg. and a pituitary LH fraction containing 1334 I.U./mg. were employed for the production of antisera.

These antisera were made specific by repeated immunoabsorption.[9] The method of Hunter and Greenwood[11] was utilized for iodination.

The sensitivity for the FSH as well as the LH assays was 0.01 ng./ml. and the precision was ±10%. The recovery of the added hormone was in the range of 95–99% in the assays, hence no correction for losses was made. Repeated determinations performed on the same plasma sample at different time intervals did not vary more than 10–15%. All results for gonadotropins were expressed as mI.U. of the 2nd International Reference Preparation-Human Menopausal Gonadotropin (2nd IRP-HMG).

The H[3]-corticosterone displacement

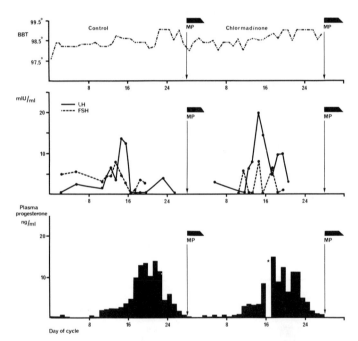

Fig. 1. Subject 1, 35 years old, Para 3, with a history of regular, 28-day cycles and an average menstrual bleeding of 3 days. The figure shows one control cycle followed by a cycle in which chlormadinone acetate, 0.5 mg., was given daily for 28 days. Upper curve shows basal body temperature (BBT), middle curve plasma levels of FSH and LH in mI.U./ml., and lower curve plasma progesterone level in ng./ml. *, days when plasma sample for progesterone determinations were not available; MP, menstrual period.

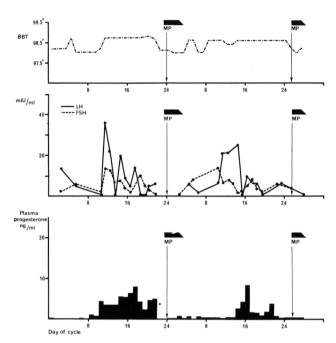

Fig. 2. Subject 2, 35 years old, Para 2, with a history of regular 28-day cycles and average menstrual flow of 4 days. For indices consult Fig. 1.

method for progesterone introduced by Murphy[12] was used with minor modifications. Binding protein was obtained from a male dog treated continuously with stilbestrol and with dexamethasone 16 hr. prior to venipuncture. The assays were performed on 0.25-ml. or 0.50-ml. plasma samples, and labeled progesterone was used for control of recovery, which was 90–95%. Under our assay conditions the sensitivity was 0.2 ng. of progesterone/ml. Repeated determination of the same sample, kept in the freezer and thawed immediately before performing the assay, gave a variation of ±12%.

RESULTS

The patterns of plasma FSH, LH, and progesterone as well as the BBT in the 9 patients are shown in Figs. 1–9.

Patient 1. Rising levels of LH over 4 days were observed from Day 11, but peak values were obtained on Days 15 and 16 (13.5 and 12.5 mI.U./ml.) (Fig. 1). Plasma progesterone values of 2–3 ng./ml. were detectable from Day 11, but a rapid rise occurred from Day 17 to a peak level (13–14 ng./ml.) on Days 19–22. Even though the increase in the BBT was not particularly clear, the pattern of LH and progesterone suggested that ovulation had taken place in the control cycle. In the chlormadinone cycle an increase in plasma LH on Day 13 (6.5 mI.U./ml.) and a peak value on Day 15 (20 mI.U./ml.) were observed. This rise in LH was associated with an increase in plasma progesterone on Day 12 (2.1 ng./ml.) and with elevated values on Days 18–23 (10.0 ng.–12.0 ng./ml.). The LH and progesterone curves in the chlormadinone

81

cycle were considered indicative of ovulation and this was further supported by a biphasic temperature curve. It is of interest that the FSH level remained relatively low in both cycles, even though a small increase was seen 1 day before the LH peak in the control cycle.

Patient 2 (Fig. 2). A peak value for LH was evident on Day 12 (33.0 mI.U./ml.) in the control cycle. Two additional LH peaks of smaller size were observed on Days 15 and 18. The first elevated progesterone value (4.5 ng./ml.) was observed on Day 11 and the elevation persisted for 11 days. The occurrence of ovulation in the control cycle was supported by the LH and progesterone patterns and also by a biphasic BBT. In the chlormadinone cycle the LH curve was characterized by three elevated midcycle values. Even though these LH values were compatible with ovulation, the progesterone level remained relatively low and the basal body temperature did not show a midcycle rise.

Patient 3. An increase in the LH level was observed as early as Days 11 and 12 in the control cycle (Fig. 3). The significance of this early rise in LH remains obscure particularly since it was not associated with any rise in plasma progesterone. On Day 16 a distinct LH peak was observed (16.5 mI.U./ml.). The progesterone began to increase on Day 17, and reached peak values on Days 20 and 21 (12.7 and 13.2 ng./ml.). The LH and progesterone patterns were considered ovulatory. The basal body temperature curve showed a slight increase at the time when ovulation was considered to have taken place. In the chlormadinone cycle two LH peaks were observed, one on

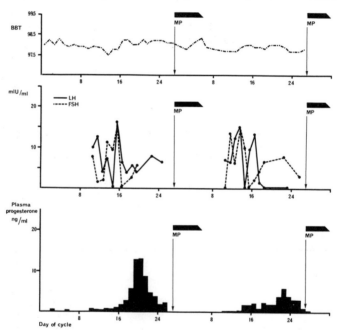

Fig. 3. Subject 3, 35 years old, Para 3, with a history of regular 28-day cycles and an average menstrual flow of 5 days. Had previous tubal ligation. For indices consult Fig. 1.

Day 14, the other on Day 17. Progesterone showed a small increase on Day 15 (2.0 ng./ml.), and then remained at a level of 2 - 6 ng./ml. for a number of days. The chlormadinone cycle was considered ovulatory even though some uncertainty exists in regard to this interpretation because of the relatively small increase in the progesterone level. It is of interest that in Patient 3 the FSH level was relatively high.

Patient 4. The plasma LH in the control cycle was high on Day 11 (23 mI.U./ml.) and fell to low levels by Day 14 (Fig. 4). Insufficient plasma for daily gonadotropin estimations was obtained in the 1st week of the cycle and therefore individual determinations separated by more than a few days are not joined by solid lines. The level of FSH was similar to that of LH. The LH

peak coincided with the onset of a rise in plasma progesterone on Day 11. A maximum was reached on Day 16 (11.5 ng./ml.) and a level of 4.5-7.8 ng./ml. was maintained until Day 21. It was considered, therefore, that ovulation occurred in the control cycle and this was supported by a midcycle rise in BBT. In the chlormadinone cycle the temperature curve was flat, the LH level fluctuated and was lower than in the control cycle. A rise in FSH to 15 mI.U./ml. was noted on Day 15. The plasma progesterone level remained low (3.4-4.4 ng./ml.) all through the cycle. The results imply that ovulation did not occur in the chlormadinone cycle.

Patient 5. LH peaks occurred on Days 12 and 17 ((the control cycle (Fig. 5). A rise in plasma progesterone was observed on

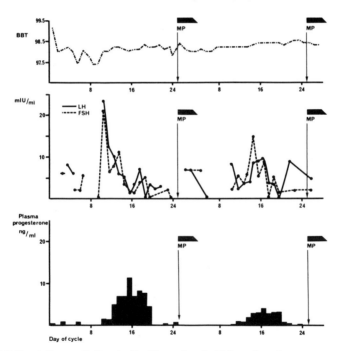

Fig. 4. Subject 4, 33 years old, Para 4, with a history of regular 26-day cycles and an average menstrual flow of 4 days. Had previous tubal ligation. For indices consult Fig. 1.

83

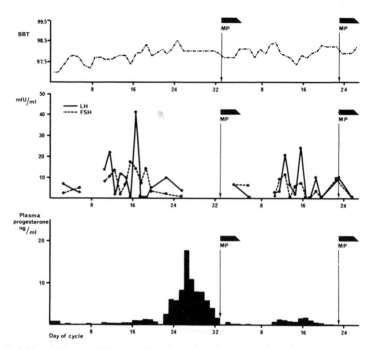

FIG. 5. Subject 5, 23 years old, Para 1, with a history of regular 28-day cycles and an average menstrual flow of 4 days. For indices consult Fig. 1.

Day 23, 5 days after the second LH peak. The presence of the LH peaks, elevated progesterone, and a biphasic BBT supported the view that ovulation had occurred. Also in the chlormadinone cycle, two LH peaks were present. The plasma progesterone remained low and the BBT was atypical. The chlormadinone cycle, therefore, was considered anovulatory.

Patient 6. The possibility of an early ovulation in the control cycle of this patient was suggested by a maximal elevation of LH (26 mI.U./ml.) on Day 8 (Fig. 6). This was coincident with a rise in progesterone also on Day 8, and a moderate progesterone level was maintained for at least 13 days. In the chlormadinone cycle, plasma levels of FSH, LH, and progesterone remained low suggesting that ovula-

tion did not occur. The biphasic BBT, however, did not support this view.

Patient 7. The control cycle was of particular interest since two LH peaks were found to be present (Fig. 7). The plasma progesterone level rose earlier than the first LH peak and also showed a biphasic pattern. The midcycle LH and progesterone levels were relatively high and the control cycle was considered ovulatory, but the exact day of ovulation was difficult to determine. In the chlormadinone cycle the double LH peak pattern was preserved to some extent, although the values were lower than in the control cycle. The progesterone level was also low. The chlormadinone cycle was regarded as nonovulatory.

Patient 8. A marked increase in the progesterone values, rising as high as 29.5

84

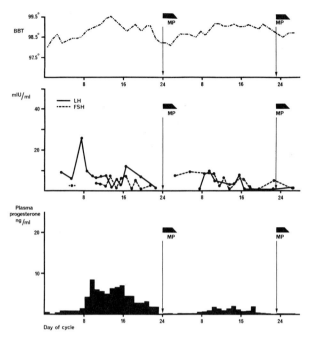

FIG. 6. Subject 6, 36 years old, no previous pregnancies with a history of regular 28-day cycles and an average menstrual flow of 7 days. For indices consult Fig. 1.

ng./ml. on Day 17, was evident in the control cycle (Fig. 8). The onset of this increase coincided with an LH peak of 15.5 m.I.U./ml. on Day 12 and a significant rise in BBT. As compared to this cycle, which was considered ovulatory, the chlormadinone cycle was regarded as nonovulatory. The LH peak values of 10 mI.U./ml. were borderline and the level of progesterone, even though reaching 6.0–8.8 ng./ml., was low in comparison with the control cycle.

Patient 9. A distinct LH peak was present in the control cycle (Fig. 9). In spite of this, ovulation was not considered to have taken place, because of the low progesterone level. Also in the chlormadinone cycle an "ovulatory" LH peak was present. A rise in progesterone occurred 6 days after the LH peak. The late appearance of

this increase and the relatively low level of progesterone makes it doubtful whether ovulation took place in this cycle. Figure 9 clearly demonstrates how difficult individual interpretation can be.

The daily mean values and the standard error (S.E.) for plasma LH and FSH are shown in Fig. 10. Day 0 represents the day of maximal plasma LH for each cycle for each patient. The mean LH value on Day 0 of the control cycle was 27.0 mI.U./ml. ± 4.0 (S.E.). The mean FSH value on Day 0 was 12.8 mI.U./ml. ± 1.9. The midcycle LH peak (16.2 mI.U./ml. ± 2.8) was more depressed in the chlormadinone cycle than FSH (9.4 mI.U./ml. ± 1.0). The plasma progesterone values covered a wide range and also appeared to be depressed during the treated cycle (Fig. 10).

In Table 1, data concerning all 9 patients have been summarized. An attempt has been made to evaluate the different curves contained in Figs. 1-9 in terms of ovulation. A midcycle LH peak of 15.0 mI.U./ml. or above was considered to be "ovulatory" for this purpose.

DISCUSSION

Only a few investigators have attempted to clarify the action of chlormadinone on ovulation. Connell[1] concluded, on the basis of endometrial biopsies in 64 normal women, that 78% appeared to have ovulated on 0.5 mg. of chlormadinone daily. Orr and Elstein[7] used parameters such as urinary LH and pregnanediol determination, as well as "spinnbarkeit" and basal body temperature to evaluate the effect of

chlormadinone on ovulation in 4 women. They found that the excretion of LH was lower than normal in 7 out of 9 cycles; however, they concluded, on the basis of the other parameters that ovulation had taken place. Jaffe and Midgley[6] studied the plasma levels of LH in 5 women, and found occasional "broad, low, abortive peaks;" only 1 woman was considered to have ovulated, as evidenced by a shift in basal body temperature and elevated urinary pregnanediol value. Recently Diczfalusy et al.[4] studied urinary LH, estrogens, and pregnanediol in 3 women during 2 control cycles and 2 chlormadinone cycles. Urinary LH peaks were absent in 5 of the 6 chlormadinone cycles.

The range of normal values for the midcycle LH peak reported in recent literature

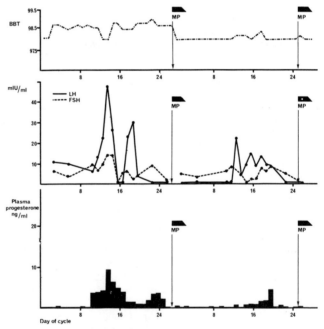

FIG. 7. Subject 7, 40 years old, no previous pregnancies with a history of regular 27-day cycles and an average menstrual flow of 7 days. For indices consult Fig. 1.

86

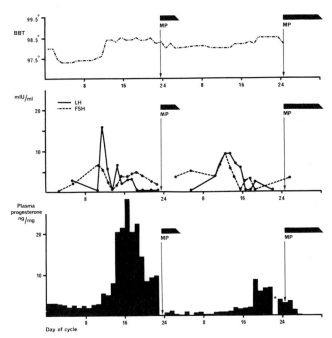

FIG. 8. Subject 8, 39 years old, Para 3, history of regular 24-day cycles and an average menstrual flow of 7 days. For indices consult Fig. 1.

are somewhat higher than those observed in our control cycles. Odell, Ross, and Rayford[13] have reported values of 40–153 mI.U./ml., Saxena, Demura, Gandy, and Peterson,[14] 67–137 mI.U./ml., Cargille, Ross, and Yoshimi,[15] 72–89 mI.U./ml., and Goebelsmann, Midgley, and Jaffe,[16] approximately 50 mI.U./ml. Our values in the control cycles ranged from 13.5–48.0 mI.U./ml. This LH assay, using pituitary LH which was available only recently, produced lower LH values than those using antibody prepared to human chorionic gonadotropin (HCG). The level of LH in the chlormadinone cycle varied considerably. Thus in Cases 1, 2, 3, and 9 the LH peaks appeared to be normal, whereas in Cases 4 and 6 the LH peaks were considerably lower than normal. The mean value

for the midcycle LH peak in the chlormadinone cycle was lower than that in the control cycle (Fig. 10).

Another finding in our study was the appearance of two clearly separated LH peaks in some control cycles and also in some chlormadinone cycles. This was particularly evident in Patient 7. At the present time the physiologic significance of two LH peaks is incompletely understood. The question of whether ovulation is initiated by the first or the second peak in these cycles remains a great challenge. Two clearly separated LH peaks in a normal, menstruating woman have been described earlier by Saxena et al.[14] and recent attention has been drawn to the occurrence of double peaks by Thomas, Walckiers, and Ferin.[17]

87

Plasma progesterone levels during the normal luteal phase have been studied extensively by many investigators,[18-20] but so far, an "ovulatory" level has not been clearly established. This may be due to the fact that the evaluation of the progesterone level involves not only the absolute values but also the number of days a certain level is maintained. It is difficult indeed, in each individual case, to evaluate one or two very high values in one cycle as compared to lower but more sustained values in another cycle. For this reason we have avoided calculating means for plasma progesterone: the composite picture, shown in Fig. 10, illustrates merely that the distribution of values in the chlormadinone cycles tends to be lower than that in the control cycles.

Diczfalusy et al.[4] reported that in some chlormadinone cycles, "ovulatory" estrogen or pregnanediol patterns were present in the urine even though midcycle urinary LH peaks could not be demonstrated. In our study, LH peaks in the plasma were not always associated with an increase in plasma progesterone. On the other hand, the plasma progesterone level was never found to be elevated in the absence of plasma LH peaks.

The obvious difficulty in a study of this type is the selection of reliable parameters to establish whether or not ovulation has occurred. It is even more difficult to assess that ovulation has taken place normally. Although, in this study, we have used generally accepted and independent parameters such as hormonal levels and BBT, the

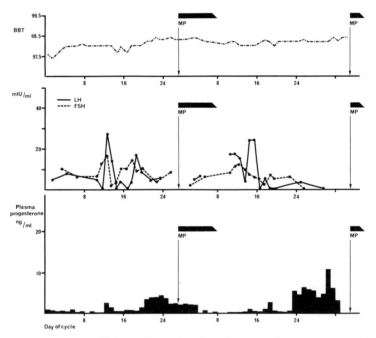

FIG. 9. Subject 9, 29 years old, Para 2, history of regular 27-day cycles and an average menstrual flow of 6 days. For indices consult Fig. 1.

88

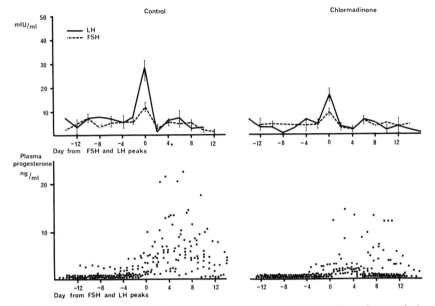

FIG. 10. Composite data of FSH, LH, and progesterone values during control and chlormadinone cycles in the nine women studied. Mean values ± S.E. (standard error) of FSH and LH are shown. On the graph the peak value of LH represents Day 0. For indices consult Fig. 1.

TABLE 1. Composite Picture of Three Different Parameters in the Nine Patients Interpreted as Positive (+) or Negative (−) from Curves Presented in Figs. 1–9

Patient no.	Control cycle			Chlormadinone cycle		
	Basal body temperature*	FSH and LH peak†	Progesterone peak‡	Basal body temperature*	FSH and LH peak†	Progesterone peak‡
1	+	+	+	+	+	+
2	+	+	+	−	+	+
3	+	+	+	−	+	+
4	+	+	+	−	−	−
5	+	+	+	−	+	−
6	+	+	+	+	−	−
7	−	+	+	−	+	−
8	+	+	+	−	−	−
9	−	+	−	−	+	−

* Basal body temperature: +, biphasic curve; −, monophasic curve.
† FSH and LH peak: +, ovulatory; −, nonovulatory.
‡ Progesterone: +, ovulatory; −, nonovulatory.

interpretation of the different curves as shown in Figs. 1–9 has required empirical decisions in borderline cases. It seems however, that in spite of limitations of the above parameters, long-term studies of the effect of chlormadinone have to be performed along these lines, since other direct evidence of ovulation, such as pregnancy or the direct observation of a corpus luteum, have limited applicability.

According to Table 1, eight of the nine women in our study ovulated in the control cycle as judged by three parameters. In the chlormadinone cycle one woman (Patient 1) ovulated by three parameters. Patients 2 and 3 ovulated by the LH and progesterone parameters, even though the levels of progesterone were not as high as in their control cycles. The low level of plasma progesterone suggests the possibility that although ovulation took place during the chlormadinone cycle in Patients 2 and 3, the subsequent low progesterone levels were produced by a poorly developed corpus luteum. It indicates the existence of an "inadequate luteal phase," further substantiated by the flat BBT curves.

The findings in this investigation, and by others previously, indicate that daily administration of 0.5 mg. of chlormadinone suppressed ovulation in some women but not in others. Whether this means that an entirely normal ovulation can take place when chlormadinone is given is not exactly known. It would appear that this question cannot be answered until the different phases of ovulation can be studied in more detail.

Rudel[21] has attempted to define the minimum contraceptive dosage of chlormadinone. He found that 0.25 mg. daily began to reduce the contraceptive effectiveness. Theoretically one would expect ovulation to take place more frequently at a dosage of chlormadinone lower than 0.5 mg. daily. It is an interesting question whether the introduction of more ovulatory cycles, by lowering the dose to 0.3 mg. or 0.4 mg. daily, would also result in a decrease in known side effects of chlormadinone, such as cycle irregularity.

SUMMARY

Nine women were studied in 1 control cycle and 1 cycle in which chlormadinone 0.5 mg. was administered daily. Plasma FSH and LH, plasma progesterone, and basal body temperature were followed. The
assessment of the individual parameters in each case was at times difficult because of the considerable variation in hormone patterns in the individual patients. A careful interpretation of the results obtained from the different parameters made us conclude that eight out of nine women ovulated in the control cycles and that three out of nine women ovulated in the chlormadinone cycles. The mean LH and FSH peaks and the plasma progesterone level in the chlormadinone cycles were found to be suppressed.

Acknowledgments. We would like to acknowledge the helpful advice given to us by George Wilson, Clinical Research Unit, Maternity Hospital, Aberdeen, Scotland, and the excellent technical assistance of Mrs. Georgianna Guzman, Miss Ingvor Jonsson, and Miss Marjorie Medina.

REFERENCES

1. CONNELL, E. B. "Daily Low Dosage Chlormadinone Administration for Conception Control. Advances in Planned Parenthood." In *Excerpta Medica Int Cong Ser 138*, Amsterdam, 1966, p. 74.
2. MARTINEZ-MANAUTOU, J., CORTEZ, V., GINER, J., AZNAR, R., CASASOLA, J., AND RUDEL, H. W. Low doses of progestogen as an approach to fertility control. *Fertil Steril 17:*49, 1966.
3. MARTINEZ-MANAUTOU, J., GINER-VELASQUEZ, J., CORTES-GALLEGOS, V., AZNAR, R., ROJAS, B., GUTEREZ-NAJAR, A., AND RUDEL, H. W. Daily progestogen for contraception: a clinical study. *Brit Med J 2:*730, 1967.
4. DICZFALUSY, E., GOEBELSMANN, U., JOHANNISSON, E., TILLINGER, K.-G., AND WIDE, L. Pituitary and ovarian function in women on continuous low dose progestogens: Effect of chlormadinone acetate and norethisterone. *Acta Endocr (Kobenhavn) 62:*679, 1969.
5. FOSS, G. L., SVENDSEN, E. K., FOTHERBY, K., AND RICHARDS, D. J. Contraceptive action of continuous low doses of norgestrel. *Brit Med J 4:*489, 1968.
6. JAFFE, R. B., AND MIDGLEY, A. R., JR. Current status of human gonadotropin radioimmunoassay. *Obstet Gynec Survey 24:*200, 1969.
7. ORR, A. H., AND ELSTEIN, M. Luteinizing hormone levels in plasma and urine in women during normal menstrual cycles and in women taking

combined contraceptives or chlormadinone acetate. *J Endocr 43:*617, 1969.

8. RATHNAM, P., AND SAXENA, B. B. Isolation and physico-chemical characterization of LH from human pituitaries. *J Biol Chem*. In press, 1970.

9. SAXENA, P. B., LEYENDECKER, G., CHEN, W., GANDY, H. M., AND PETERSON, R. E. Radioimmunoassay of follicle stimulating (FSH) and luteinizing (LH) hormones by chromatoelectrophoresis. *Acta endocr 63 (Suppl 142):*185, 1969.

10. SAXENA, B. B., AND RATHNAM, P. Purification of follicle-stimulating hormone from human pituitary glands. *J Biol Chem 242:*3769, 1967.

11. HUNTER, W. M., AND GREENWOOD, F. C. Preparation of I¹³¹ labelled human growth hormone of high specific activity. *Nature (London) 194:*495, 1962.

12. MURPHY, B. E. P. Some studies of the protein-binding of steroid and their application to the routine micro and ultramicro measurement of various steroids in body fluids by competitive protein-binding radioassay. *J Clin Endocr 27:*973, 1967.

13. ODELL, W. D., ROSS, G. T., AND RAYFORD, P. L. Radioimmunoassay for luteinizing hormone in human plasma or serum: Physiological studies. *J Clin Invest 46:*248, 1967.

14. SAXENA, B. B., DEMURA, H., GANDY, H. M., AND PETERSON, R. E. Radioimmunoassay of human follicle-stimulating and luteinizing hormone in plasma. *J Clin Endocr 28:*519, 1968.

15. CARGILLE, C. M., ROSS, G. T., AND YOSHIMI, T. Daily variation in plasma follicle-stimulating hormone, luteinizing hormone and progesterone in the normal menstrual cycle. *J Clin Endocr 29:* 12, 1969.

16. GOEBELSMANN, U., MIDGLEY, A. R. JR., AND JAFFE, R. B. Regulation of human gonadotropins. VII. Daily individual urinary estrogens, pregnanediol and serum luteinizing and follicle-stimulating hormones during the menstrual cycle. *J Clin Endocr 29:*1222, 1969.

17. THOMAS, K., WALCKIERS, R., AND FERIN, J. Biphasic pattern of LH mid-cycle discharge. *J Clin Endocr 30:*269, 1970.

18. NEILL, J. D., JOHANSSON, E. D. B., DATTA, J. K., AND KNOBIL, E. Relationship between the plasma levels of luteinizing hormone and progesterone during the normal menstrual cycle. *J Clin Endocr 27:*1167, 1967.

19. VAN DER MOLEN, H. J., AND GROEN, D. Determination of progesterone in human peripheral blood using gas-liquid chromatography with electron capture detection. *J Clin Endocr 25:*1625, 1965.

20. YOSHIMI, T., AND LIPSETT, M. B. The measurement of plasma progesterone. *Steroids 11:*527, 1968.

21. RUDEL, H. W. "Hormonal Fertility Control—Newer Biological Consideration." In *Excerpta Medica Int Congr Ser 133*, Amsterdam, 1967, p. 994.

Histologic Study of the Uterine Cervix During Oral Contraception with Ethynodiol Diacetate and Mestranol

EMILIO CARBIA, MD, FACS, GUILLERMO RUBIO-LINARES, MD, ALBERTO ALVARADO-DURAN, MD, and MARIO LOPEZ-LLERA, MD

THE EXTENSIVE USE of synthetic steroids for contraception and a variety of gynecologic disorders has created growing concern and extensive controversy about their immediate and long-term effects. Of special importance is the possible carcinogenic influence of these drugs in the cervical epithelium. Some recent clinical and experimental reports seem to indicate that the estrogen-progestogen combinations do not have any apparent carcinogenic effect when used in therapeutic doses.

Kaminetzky studied the changes produced by sex steroids on 3-methylcholanthrene-induced squamous cell atypia of the uterine cervix and vagina of castrated mice; he concluded that progesterone appears to counteract the tendency of estrogen to induce stromal penetration by dysplastic cells. Tóth and Szónyi tested the effect of a synthetic steroid in rats with induced tumors; they found a reduction in the number of mitoses and a prolongation of the latent period of tumor formation, indicating that the drug had an antineoplastic effect. Pincus[13] presented data showing the prevalence of suspicious vaginal smears and cervical biopsies among users of oral steroid contraceptives in comparison with patients using spermaticides or intrauterine devices. In the group taking oral contraceptives, there was a lower frequency of suspicious smears and cervical biopsies suggesting a preventive effect of the steroids. Pincus and Garcia[5, 14] also stated that there is evidence that the incidence of potential precancerous conditions of the endometrium, the cervix, and the breasts is reduced in oral contraceptive users, and that there is no direct evidence to suggest a carcinogenic potential of these agents. Loraine and Bell are of the same opinion. Brehm and Käser using colposcopy and cytologic smears found no sign of the presence of cervical carcinoma in patients taking these drugs. Wied and associates compared the cytologic records of 1628 patients who received hormonal contraceptives for more than 1 year with a control group of women not known to be receiving the medication; no statistically significant increase of even slightly atypia was found. Diddle, *et al* found no increase in the incidence of carcinoma in situ after as long as 6 years of oral contraception, and Rock said that after 10 years of widespread use of these substances there is no evidence of any relationship with cancer, and that plentiful data strongly suggest that, if there is any relationship, it is a favorable one.

Aside from the problem of a possible carcinogenic influence, the steroid combinations produce some other changes in the cervix that have not been well studied, and that may be of importance as contributing factors for their contraceptive action or may cause bothersome symptoms to the patients. Maqueo and associates studied the cervix of women receiving estrogen-progestogen combinations or who were treated continuously with progestational steroids—apparently no control studies were done and the comparison was made with groups of pregnant and nonpregnant women. They found hyperplasia and hypersecretion of the cervical glands, stromal edema, and squamous metaplasia, but there were no important epithelial changes. Ryan, Craig, and Reid made histologic studies of specimens from 27 patients who underwent hysterectomy after cyclic norethynodrel therapy and except for hypersecretory glands no other change was noted.

This paper reports part of a study using calposcopic, cytologic, and histologic technics to examine the uterine cervix in women being treated with an estrogen-progestogen combination. It is hoped that it may contribute in some way to the knowledge of the effects of these substances upon the cervix.

MATERIALS AND METHODS

The study was carried out in a group of patients selected at random that had been receiving oral ethynodiol diacetate and me-stranol (Ovulen, 1.0/0.1 mg)* in our Hospital.

Before oral contraception was begun, each patient underwent a complete physical examination—including cytologic smear, colposcopic observation, and cervical biopsy. These studies were repeated at intervals of 6 to 12 months, according to the availability of the patients. Whenever possible the biopsy was taken at more or less the same site as the original one, depending on the colposcopic picture and the continous movements of the cervical epithelium, giving preference to the so-called transformation zone. Cultures of the cervico-vaginal exudates were carried out in specific cases, and local treatment with vaginal tablets or superficial electrocoagulation was given when necessary. The latter was not performed until the patients had been 6–12 months under medication with the oral contraceptive; the cervical biopsy was obtained before electrocoagulation and not repeated until another 6–12 months had elapsed. The contraceptive medication was given according to the cyclic method. The histologic studies were done with the usual technic for conventional light microscopy.

RESULTS

A total of 58 patients had repeated cervical biopsies for histologic study under colposcopic control. The age of the patients varied from 20 to 43 years with an average of 30.9 years; more than half of them were in the age groups between 30 to 39 or over 40 years, with a high average number of previous gestations (Table 1). In 44 of the 58 patients the pretreatment control biopsy was obtained 1–3 months after the end of pregnancy (Table 2). Eight patients had their first control biopsy taken between 6 and 11 months of medication, 22 patients had one or two biopsies taken between 12 and 23 months, and 28 patients were stud-

* G. D. Searle & Company, Chicago, Ill 60680.

93

TABLE 1. DISTRIBUTION OF PATIENTS BY AGE AND PREVIOUS GESTATIONS

	Age		
	20–29	30–39	> 40
No. of patients	24 (41.4%)	28 (48.3%)	6 (10.3%)
Previous pregnancies (Average No.)	4.8	7.7	11.6

TABLE 2. TIME BETWEEN END OF PREGNANCY AND PRETREATMENT BIOPSY

Outcome of pregnancy	Months				No. of patients
	1	1–3	3–6	>6	
Delivery or cesarean section	7	25	3	4	39
Abortion	1	6	—	—	7
Hydatidiform mole	1	4	6	1	12
TOTAL	9	35	9	5	58

ied with repeated biopsies during 24–40 months of uninterrupted treatment with the synthetic steroids (Table 3). Three patients had been suspected of having carcinoma in situ of the cervix during pregnancy, but this was not proven after delivery. Seven patients had a biopsy taken 1–6 months after the medication was discontinued to serve as post-treatment controls. Another 4 patients, who were pregnant before or after the steroids were given, also had cervical biopsies. Altogether a total of 181 histologic examinations were done.

The histologic findings in the ectocervical epithelium are summarized in Table 4. As it can be seen, parakeratosis was already present in 35 patients before treatment began; it appeared for the first time during

TABLE 3. DURATION OF TREATMENT AND NO. OF BIOPSIES STUDIED

	Duration of treatment (months)			
	6–11	12–23	24–35	35–40
No. of patients	8	22	22	6
No. of biopsies	8	36	50	18
Average No. of biopsies	1	1.6	2.2	3

medication in 16 patients and it was not observed again in 7 of these (Fig 1). Together with parakeratosis, a thickening of the epithelium was noted in 17 patients. Basal cell hyperplasia and slight or focal dysplasia were present before treatment in 10 patients, but in 9 of them they were not observed again during medication. These changes were found for the first time during the administration of the drug in 5 women, but they were not reflected in the cytologic smear or at colposcopy. Parakeratosis persisted in the 7 patients who had a post-treatment biopsy, and in 1 patient moderate dysplasia was reported 1 month after the steroids had been discontinued.

During all the time of uninterrupted medication, colposcopy did not show suspicious zones in any of the patients and cytologic reports were consistently negative, showing only inflammatory changes. In a single patient the cytologic smear was reported as suspicious, but after treatment of the cervicovaginal infection it became negative and has remained so.

The most conspicuous changes occurred in the glandular structures and stroma (Table 4). In most patients there was an increase in size and number of the glands, sometimes with irregular shape and invagination and papillary formations of the epithelium (Fig 2 and 3). Also, in most cases, the glands showed signs of active secretion of mucus during medication. In 15 specimens these changes were classified as adenomatous hyperplasia. One endocervical polyp became larger, edematous, and with signs of vascular congestion. Squamous metaplasia persisted in 4 of the original pa-

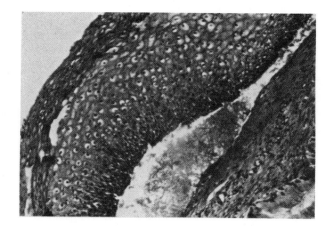

Fig 1. Persistence of superficial cornified layer or parakeratosis, and thickening of ectocervical epithelium, with basal cell hyperplasia and inflammatory reaction. (H&E, × 50)

tients and it was observed in another 18 during treatment (Fig 4). There was an increase in the vascularization in more than half of the biopsies studied; the blood vessels were mainly capillaries, but in 10, a thickening of their walls at the expense of the muscular layer was found (Fig 5). The intensity of acute and chronic inflammatory reaction also increased in many instances (Fig 6); sometimes it was found focally

TABLE 4. HISTOLOGIC FINDINGS IN THE ECTOCERVICAL EPITHELIUM, ENDOCERVICAL GLANDS, AND STROMA

Histologic findings before medication	No.	Without change	First observed	Not observed again	Increase Moderate	Marked
ECTOCERVICAL EPITHELIUM						
Normal	21	7	—	—	—	—
Parakeratosis	35	18	16	7	10	—
Thickening	5	5	17	—	—	—
Basal cell hyperplasia	5	1	3	4	—	—
Slight or focal dysplasia	5	—	2	5	—	—
ENDOCERVICAL GLANDS*						
Normal amount	35	7	—	—	10	18
Increased amount	19	1	—	—	8	10
Signs of secretion	23	8	31	—	11	4
Squamous metaplasia	6	4	18	2	—	—
STROMA						
Vascularization						
Normal	29	3	—	—	18	8
Increased	29	16	—	—	13	—
Inflammatory reaction						
Slightly increased	18	2	—	—	9	7
Moderately increased	20	7	—	—	10	3
Markedly increased	20	16	—	—	3	—

* In 4 patients endocervical glands could not be studied.

95

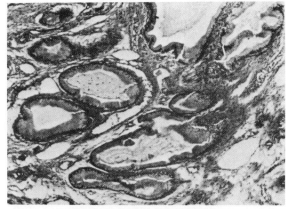

Fig 2. Endocervical glands of different sizes, slightly irregular and with signs of active secretion. (H&E, × 50)

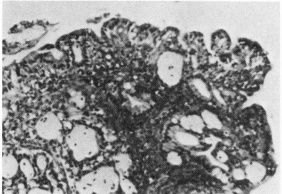

Fig 3. Abundant endocervical glands of different sizes. Endocervical epithelium shows tendency to form papillary formations. (H&E, × 25)

around the glands, and at other times, diffuse and intense. No stromal edema or decidual reaction was observed, but in some cases there was a tendency to fibrosis. In 6 of the 7 patients who had a control biopsy after treatment, the glands diminished in size and number, with less vascularization and diminished inflammatory reaction of the stroma. In contrast, the biopsies taken during pregnancy showed glandular hyperplasia, signs of active secretion, and squamous metaplasia, together with increased vascularization, inflammatory reaction, and edema of the stroma.

COMMENT

The histologic findings during treatment with ethynodiol diacetate and mestranol show close correlation with the colposcopic changes of the cervix reported by Carbia, Lopez-Llera, and Alvarado-Duran. These consist of an increase in size of the area of ectopia and ectropion with a tendency of the endocervical epithelium to show polypoid formations, an increased vascularization and a greater quantity of mucus.

The fact that no special epithelial changes were found during treatment with sex steroids in a group of patients with an average

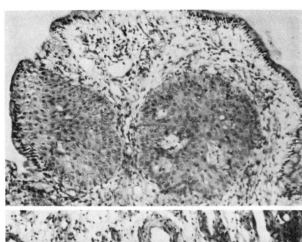

Fig 4. Squamous metaplasia. (H&E, × 100)

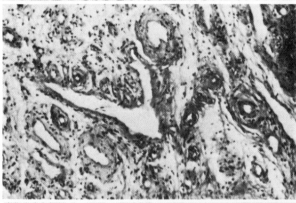

Fig 5. Blood vessels with thickened walls, some times at expense of muscular layer. (H&E, × 100)

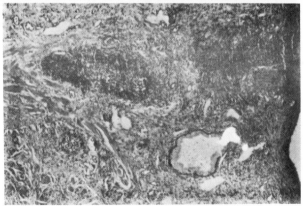

Fig 6. Diffuse and intense chronic inflammatory reaction in stroma. (H&E, × 100)

age of 30.9 years, a high number of previous gestations, and a low socioeconomic condition seems important, although as Hertz and Bailar pointed out, they have not been followed for a suitable period of time. Nevertheless, there is complete disagreement with the report of Guhr, who studied 65 patients who had been taking ovulation inhibitors for several years, for he found definite histologic changes, ranging through parakeratosis in 100% of the patients, proliferation of the basal squamous epithelium in 64%, and findings suggesting surface carcinoma in 11%. On the other hand our work tends to support Ayre and associates who have been studying the effects of norethynodrel and mestranol upon inflammatory, precancerous lesions and carcinoma in situ of the cervix; they concluded that the outstanding result of their study was the abscence of any tangible or recognizable change to indicate accelerated progression of dysplastic or neoplastic epithelium during prolonged periods of steroid medication. Furthermore, parakeratosis, glandular changes, squamous metaplasia, increased vascularization, and inflammatory reaction are found in many patients not taking steroids, findings that in most instances seem to depend upon the particular area of the cervix biopsied and upon the presence of infection. According to Hellman and to Moore and Taylor these histologic changes are common during pregnancy, especially dysplasia of the ectocervical epithelium, reserve cell hyperplasia, squamous metaplasia, and glandular hyperplasia with signs of active secretion. Since more than half of the patients in this study had the pretreatment control biopsy 1–3 months after delivery or abortion, many of the histologic changes could represent a remaining effect. It is possible that treatment with the estrogen-progestogen medication provided enough stimulus for their persistence. The fact that the quantity of glands, the intensity of the vascularization, and the inflammatory reaction diminished in the post-treatment biopsies, in contrast with the findings during pregnancy, seems to substantiate this impression.

Although it is difficult to draw any definite conclusion from the study of the small amount of tissue obtained with a biopsy, even under colposcopic guidance, our impression is that long-term oral contraception with ethynodiol diacetate and mestranol does cause some cervical changes similar to, but less marked than those found during pregnancy. These changes may enhance the contraceptive action, but also, mimicking the pregnant condition, they may increase the clinical importance and the corresponding microscopic findings of common pre-existent benign cervical lesions, such as acute and chronic cervicitis, ectopia, ectropion, polyps, etc. Consequently, the cervix must be thoroughly examined and treated, if necessary, before starting oral contraception—more so if an oral contraceptive is to be prescribed shortly after delivery.

REFERENCES

1. AYRE, J. E., HILLEMANNS, H. G., LE GUER-RIER, J., et al. Influence of norethynodrel and mestranol upon cervical dysplasia and carcinoma in situ. *Obstet Gynec 28:*90, 1966.

2. BREHM, H., and KÄSER, O. New facts on short and long term administration of hormonal contraceptives. *Excerpta Medica Foundation International Congress Series 130:*102, 1966.

3. CARBIA, E., LOPEZ-LLERA, M., and ALVARADO-DURAN, A. Colposcopic study of the uterine cervix during the administration of ethynodiol diacetate with mestranol. *Amer J Obstet Gynec 102:*1023, 1968.

4. DIDDLE, A. W., WATTS, G. F., GARDNER, W. H., et al. Oral contraceptive medication. A prolonged experience. *Amer J Obstet Gynec 95:*489, 1966.

5. GARCIA, C. R., and PINCUS, G. Clinical considerations of oral hormonal control of human fertility. *Clin Obstet Gynec 7:*844, 1964.

6. GUHR, VON G. Bietrag über die Wirkung von Ovulationshemmern auf das Plattenepithel der portio Uteri. *Z Geburtsh Gynaek 88:*815, 1966.

7. HELLMAN, L. M. "Changes in Cervical Epithelium During Pregnancy." In *Progress in Gynecology,* (Vol. III), Meigs, J. V., and Sturgis, S. H., Eds. Grune, New York–London, 1957, p 433.

8. HERTZ, R., and BAILAR, J. C. Estrogen-progestogen combinations for contraception. *JAMA 198:*136, 1966.

9. KAMINETZKY, H. A. Methylcholanthene—induced cervical dysplasia and the sex steroids. *Obstet Gynec 27:*489, 1966.

10. LORAINE, J. A., and BELL, E. T. *Fertility and Contraception in the Human Female,* Livingstone, Edinburgh and London, 1968, p 277.

11. MAQUEO, M., AZUELA, J. CH., CALDERON, J. J., et al. Morphology of the cervix in women treated with synthetic pregestins. *Amer J Obstet Gynec 96:*994, 1966.

12. MOORE, D. B., and TAYLOR, H. C. "The Pregnancy Problem." In *Dysplasia, Carcinoma in situ and Microinvasive—Carcinoma of the Cervix Uteri,* Gray, L. A., Ed. Charles C Thomas, Springfield, Ill, 1964, p 256.

13. PINCUS, G. *The Control of Fertility.* Acad. Press, New York–London, 1965, p 256.

14. PINCUS, G., and GARCIA, C. R. "Long–Term Use of Progestin–Oestrogen Combinations." In *Recent Advances in Ovarian Synthetic Steroids and the Control of Ovarian Function,* Shearman, R. P., Ed. G. D. Searle & Co. Ltd., Sidney, 1965, p 104.

15. ROCK, J. "Oral Contraceptives." In *The Year Book of Obstetrics and Gynecology,* Greenhill, J. P., Ed. Year Book Medical Publishers, Chicago, 1966–1967, p 398.

16. RYAN, G. M., CRAIG, J., and REID, D. E. Histology of the uterus and ovaries after long-term cyclic norethynodrel therapy. *Amer J Obstet Gynec 90:*715, 1964.

17. TÓTH, F., and SZÓNYI, I. The inhibiting effect of a norsteroid on tumor formation and the metabolism of tumor cells. *Amer J Obstet Gynec 94:*518, 1966.

18. WIED, G. L., DAVIS, M. E., FRANK, R., et al. Statistical evaluation of the effect of hormonal contraceptives on the cytological smear pattern. *Obstet Gynec 27:*327, 1966.

99

Endometrial changes in women receiving oral contraceptives

JOSEPH SONG, M.D.

MILTON S. MARK, M.D.

MATTHEW P. LAWLER, JR., M.D.

ATYPICAL endocervical hyperplasia, associated with contraceptive pills, has been reported with increasing frequency in recent years and has received growing attention. According to Govan, Black, and Sharp,[1] Pincus[2] appears to have been the first to suggest that oral contraceptive pills might have a considerable effect on cervical function. This was reiterated by Greenblatt[3] in 1959, and in 1964 Zanartu[4] described a progestational-like change in the cervix of women taking the oral contraceptive pill.

Taylor, Irey, and Norris,[5] in 1967, reported on atypical endocervical hyperplasia in thirteen patients taking oral contraceptives. Fifteen cases of aberrant polypoidal glandular hyperplasia of the cervix were described in 1969 by Govan, Black, and Sharp,[1] who also found a similar lesion in 5 pregnant patients. Their remaining 10 patients had taken contraceptive pills over a considerable period of time. Govan, Black, and Sharp[1] felt that the lesion, while histologically bizarre, is benign, the changes being, to a great extent, cytoplasmic and not nuclear. Furthermore, according to Govan, Black, and Sharp,[1] the lesion was formed by the influence of steroids on the cervix. Clinical evaluation of the pelvis, Papanicolaou smears, and histologic review of cervical biopsy specimens in 103 patients were studied by Gall, Bourgeois, and Maguire[6] to evaluate the morphologic effects of oral

Supported in part by a research grant from the Iowa Division of the American Cancer Society.

contraceptive agents on the cervix. None of 103 patients taking various oral contraceptive pills showed carcinoma, but a clinical lesion was present in 84 per cent of their patients. Atypical polypoid hyperplasia of the endocervix and adenomatous hyperplasia were frequently seen in the biopsy specimens.

It is conceivable that the endometrial stroma, a pleuripotential mesodermal derivative from which the human endocervix seems to derive, may be influenced by a variety of oral contraceptive agents, if taken for a significant period of time. The present study was undertaken to review morphologic changes of the endometrium, presumably induced by oral contraceptive pills.

Material and methods

The study group consisted of 105 women taking a variety of contraceptive pills for periods ranging from 2 to 60 months: norethynodrel, 2.5 mg., mestranol, 0.1 mg. (Enovid-E), 6 women; norethindrone, 2 mg., mestranol, 0.10 mg. (Ortho-Novum), 27 women; ethynodiol diacetate, 1 mg., mestranol, 0.1 mg. (Ovulen), 25 women; ethinyl estradiol, 0.1 mg., dimethisterone, 25 mg. (Oracon), 12 women; mestranol, 0.08 mg., chlormadinone acetate, 2 mg. (C-Quens), 17 women; medroxyprogesterone acetate, 10 mg., ethinyl estradiol, 0.05 mg. (Provest), 10 women; norethindrone acetate, 2.5 mg., ethinyl estradiol, 0.05 mg. (Norlestrin), 8 women.

The patients' ages ranged from 18 to 49 years, with parity varying from 0 to 7.

Papanicolaou smears were taken and examined from all patients. Endometrial biopsies were performed in different menstrual cycles in 21 patients. Eighty-four patients were admitted for dilatation and curettage, primarily for metromenorrhagia, and 18 patients underwent subsequent hysterectomy. The cytohistologic correlation was routinely attempted, and multiple sections were prepared from each specimen for hematoxylin and eosin, Gomori's reticulum, Masson's trichrome, and Verhoeff's elastic tissue stains.

Results

For the purpose of morphologic descriptions of the endometrial changes, two major morphologic alterations are subdivided into glandular changes and stromal alterations, although these two components are inseparable, both being of Müllerian ductal origin, a derivative of the mesoderm.

Endometrial glandular changes. Examination of 12 endometrial biopsy specimens taken during the mid and late stages of proliferative phase disclosed that in 6 women the endometrial glands were generally atrophic, having small and straight glands, with minimum pseudostratification of nuclei, showing sharp contrast to marked pseudostratification of glandular cells seen in normal late proliferative endometrium. The nuclei of the glandular cells were considerably dissociated, their pseudostratification being strikingly diminished. Some of the glands were separated from the basement membrane of the stroma, having a large tissue artifact which was probably due to a sudden shrinkage of the glandular elements. Occasionally the glandular cells were markedly vacuolated, containing nuclear masses simulating a so-called Arias-Stella phenomenon. However, the Ortho immunologic pregnancy test was negative in all cases. Of 9 biopsy specimens obtained during the secretory phase, 3 endometria revealed marked atrophic changes of the glands, with no discernible subnuclear vacuolation. The surrounding stroma was quite dense, showing pronounced decidual changes, with multiple thrombosed capillaries. There was a moderate degree of adenomatous hyperplasia associated with pronounced myometrial hyperplasia in a 40-year-old woman who had had bleeding continuously after taking Oracon for 18 months.

Stromal alterations. The stromal changes observed in 26 of 105 women were generally striking.

Stromal nodular hyperplasia. The endometrium of a 32-year-old woman who had been taking C-Quens for approximately 8 months showed a marked nodular hyper-

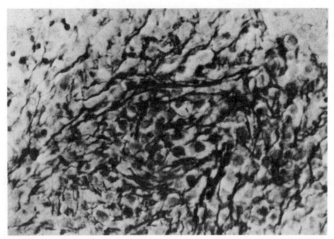

Fig. 1. Increased endometrial stromal reticulum fibers in a 32-year-old woman (C-Quens, 8 months).

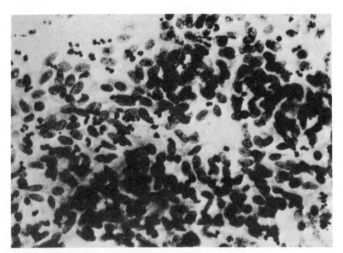

Fig. 2. Vaginal smears filled with stromal cells—same patient.

plasia of the stroma, which showed considerable proliferation of reticulum fibers seen on Gomori's reticulum stain (Fig. 1). The cervical smear previously examined disclosed a large number of endometrial stromal cells of fibroblastic type, which were quite abundant (Fig. 2).

Stromal vascularity. In a densely proliferated stroma with several small and atrophic glands there were multiple capillaries, many distended lymphatics, and numerous microcysts which were readily demonstrable. Some of the capillaries were thrombosed, while others were extremely distended, forming

102

multiple sinuses, which were likewise thrombosed (Figs. 3 and 4). The proliferation of the arteriolar walls in the endometrium was quite pronounced in the group of women taking Ovulen, Ortho-Novum, and C-Quens, showing massive proliferation of smooth muscular cells of the arterioles, with subsequent obliteration of the lumina, resulting in multiple small leiomyomas (Figs. 5 and 6). The arteriolar proliferation of smooth muscular fibers was seen exclusively in the endometrial stroma. Special stains indicated

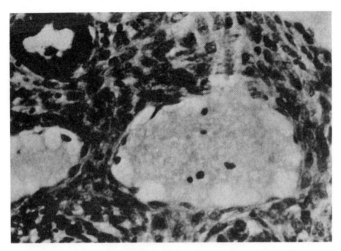

Fig. 3. Endometrium after 4 months' Ortho-Novum, showing atrophic glands and numerous capillaries and lymphatics in a 30-year-old woman.

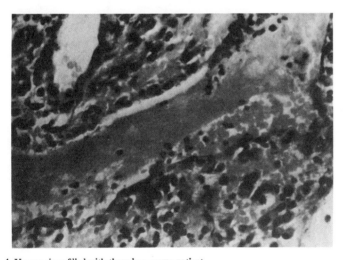

Fig. 4. Venous sinus filled with thrombus—same patient.

103

that the intimal and medial fibers were responsible for vascular proliferation, while the pericytes were uninvolved. The smooth muscle hyperplasia was frequently seen in the middle layer of the endometrium, penetrating the endometrial glands and the stroma. The distinction between the endometrial stroma and the proliferating myometrial structures was generally indistinct, suggesting the possibility of direct metaplasia from proliferating endometrial stromal cells to the muscular fibers.

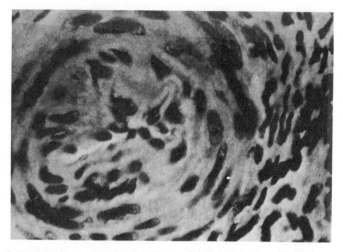

Fig. 5. Pronounced arteriolar intimal proliferation after Ortho-Novum for 6 months.

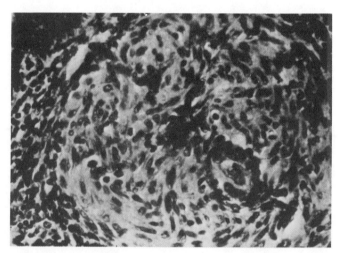

Fig. 6. Small submucous leiomyoma transformed from proliferating artery.

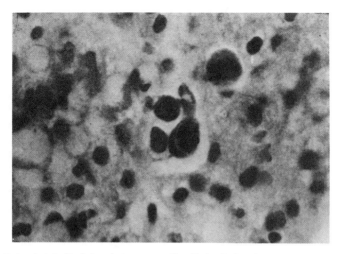

Fig. 7. Atypical decidual changes in women taking Norlestrin for 10 to 21 months.

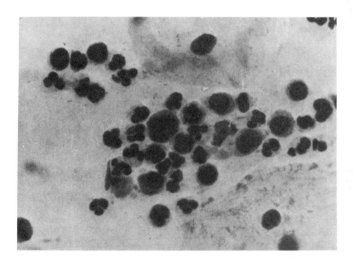

Fig. 8. Corresponding cervical smears read as suspicious epithelial cells, Class IV.

Decidual alterations. The uterine curettings obtained from women who had been taking contraceptive pills, followed by metromenorrhagia, revealed marked decidual changes of the endometrial stroma, which was frequently indistinguishable morphologically from genuine decidua. Oc-

casionally, the decidual cells were markedly atypical, having multiple mitoses and spindle-shaped, extremely hyperchromatic nuclei (Fig. 7). The cytologic examination of smears taken previously showed groups of atypical and suspicious cells, based upon which dilatation and curettage were per-

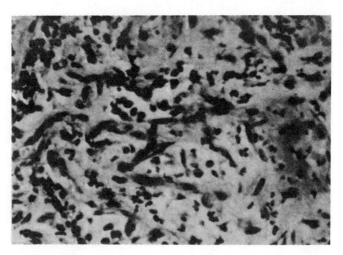

Fig. 9. Decidual changes with inflammation and hemorrhage simulating genuine decidua after Enovid-E for 19 months.

formed (Fig. 8). The endometrium of women taking Enovid-E from 13 to 17 months showed decidual changes associated with pronounced inflammation. illustrated in Fig. 9.

Anaplasia of stroma. Anaplastic changes involving the endometrial stroma were observed in 2 women who had been on Norlestrin for 33 months and Provest for 52 months, respectively. Both women were admitted for dilatation and curettage for profuse and irregular vaginal bleeding, which had occurred approximately 6 to 10 weeks prior to their admission. Multiple sections prepared from the entire specimens on both cases revealed pronounced stromal hyperplasia (Figs. 10 and 11) associated with marked anaplastic changes, as manifested by nuclear irregularities, hyperchromatic cells with prominent nucleoli, and abundant abnormal mitosis. The nuclei varied tremendously in size and shape, shedding a large number of suspicious cells examined on vaginal and cervical smears, yielding a Class IV cytologic diagnosis. Cervical conization was performed on both patients, which failed to reveal any evidence of malignant changes. Representative slides

were reviewed by several pathologists, whose impressions varied from metastatic carcinoma from the breast in the endometrium to stromal sarcoma and Müllerian duct sarcoma (Figs. 12 and 13).

Cytologic findings. The routine vaginal aspiration in cervical scraping smears examined for general female population screening procedures does not as a rule contain the endometrial stromal cells, which are readily demonstrable, unless the smears are taken during the menstrual cycle, when endometrial stromal cells possessing bean-shaped nuclei, surrounded by a scanty amount of foamy cytoplasm, may be shed from the endometrium. The most striking cytologic abnormality in the smears taken from women receiving various types of oral contraceptive agents seems to be the presence of a large number of endometrial stromal cells which are characterized by enlarged and slightly hyperchromatic nuclei with prominent nucleoli, being surrounded by an abundant yet extremely foamy pink-stained cytoplasm (Fig. 14). The nuclear membranes were frequently indented, while the staining density varied considerably from normal to marked hyperchromasia. The

106

nucleoli were generally prominent. The most characteristic cytologic finding, however, was in the cytoplasm. The foamy appearance of the cytoplasm, resulting in a fine vacuolation, with deep orange stain, exhibiting a well-outlined cell membrane, appeared to be characteristic features which would enable cytotechnologists and pathologists to distinguish stromal cells from suspicious cervical epithelial cells. The analysis of 525 smears

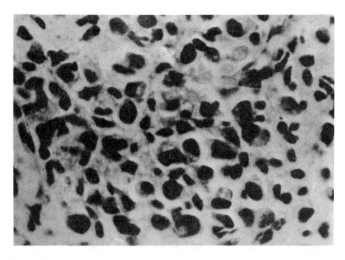

Fig. 10. Anaplastic endometrial stromal hyperplasia in a 42-year-old woman after taking Norlestrin for 33 months.

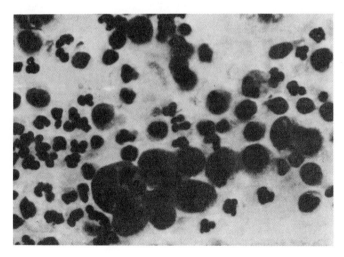

Fig. 11. Cervical smears of above patient, on whom dilatation and curettage were done, contain many suspicious cells.

107

taken from women who had been on oral contraceptive agents, and whose tissue specimens were not available for this study, showed abundant endometrial stromal cells which were subsequently identified by our cytotechnologists.

Comment

The human endometrial stroma seems to be multipotential in nature, possessing the labile character of morphologic alterations to differentiate into various components, such as endometrial glandular epithelia, stromal

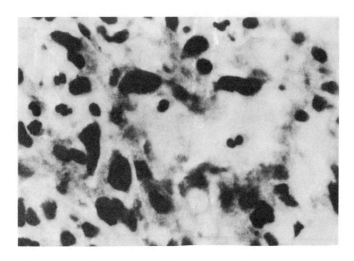

Fig. 12. Sarcomatous stromal changes in 42-year-old woman admitted for metromenorrhagia after taking Provest for 52 months.

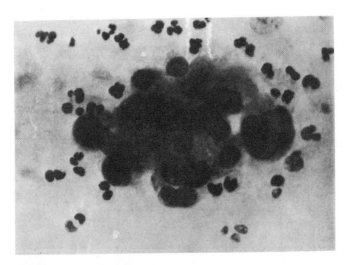

Fig. 13. Cytology, Classes IV and V. From same patient as Fig. 12.

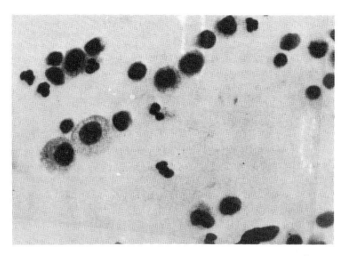

Fig. 14. Endometrial stromal cells frequently seen in routine vaginal and cervical smears taken from women taking oral contraceptives. Pleomorphic nuclei, prominent nuclei, nuclear indentations, and abundant foamy pink-colored cytoplasm.

collagen, smooth muscle fibers composing a myometrium, and endocervical stroma, from which further differentiation into the endocervical glandular epithelia takes place in the fetal uteri.[7]

Our previous observations indicated that the endometrial epithelial regeneration probably initiates from the stroma under the proper and sufficient horomonal stimuli.[7]

The oral contraceptive agents which are widely used today contain a wide variety of estrogen and progesterone in differing ratios. Progesterone has known antiestrogenic effect, but reports quoted by Gall, Bourgeois, and Maguire[6] suggested similar biologic effect attributed to progesterone and estrogen. Gall, Bourgeois, and Maguire[6] further stated that estrogen and progesterone have a specific biologic effect when administered separately, and it would seem likely that a new net effect would result when the two hormones are administered simultaneously. The net effect of the action of estrogen and progesterone would be the resultant stimulus to the endometrial stroma, which may react in a variety of ways to the differing stimuli, manifesting a pronounced decidual reaction

of the stroma, atypical decidual proliferation, glandular hyperplasia, myometrial hyperplasia, and capillary and arteriolar proliferation with thromboemboli.

The arteriolar and capillary proliferation and venous sinuses with thrombi appeared to be the manifestations of an aberrant estrogenic stimulus, since an extreme degree of serosal vascular engorgement and capillary proliferation in fetal uteri in the second trimester was thought to be due to high maternal estrogenic level.[7] The islands of hyperplastic myometrium were frequently observed in the upper portion of the endometrium, suggesting the possibility of direct metaplasia from the endometrial stroma to muscular fibers under hormonal stimuli. It is conceivable that continued application of estrogen and progesterone on the endometrial stroma would elicit anaplastic hyperplasia of stromal cells with sarcomatous changes leading into a possible neoplasm of the endometrial stroma on a sensitive individual.

It should be emphasized, however, that individual response to oral contraceptive agents seems to be extremely variable, as there were no significant morphologic changes observed in the endometria of 79 women who had been taking various oral contraceptive pills for a significant period of time. As women receive the oral contraceptive agents for greater periods of time, the endometrial stromal reaction seems to be greater, as illustrated in 2 of our cases in which anaplastic changes of stromal cells were observed. Attwood[8] recently described that progesterone increases exfoliation of abnormal cells but does not accelerate the cell beyond the halo type into maximal dysplasia. This would provide the physiologic basis for the presence of abundant endometrial stromal cells in the routine Papanicolaou smears prepared from daily patients at gynecologists' offices.

REFERENCES

1. Govan, A. D. T., Black, W. P., and Sharp, J. L.: J. Clin. Path. 22: 84, 1969.
2. Pincus, G.: Acta Endocr. (Suppl.) 28: 18, 1956.
3. Greenblatt, R. B.: Fed. Proc. 18: 1055, 1959.
4. Zanartu, J.: Int. J. Fertil. 9: 225, 1964.
5. Taylor, H. B., Irey, N. S., and Norris, H. J.: J. A. M. A. 202: 637, 1967.
6. Gall, S. A., Bourgeois, C. H., and Maguire, R.: J. A. M. A. 207: 2243, 1969.
7. Song, J.: The Human Uterus. Morphogenesis and Embryological Basis for Cancer, ed. 1, Springfield, Illinois, 1964, Charles C Thomas, Publisher.
8. Attwood, M. E.: J. Obstet. Gynaec. Brit. Comm. 73: 662, 1966.

Discussion

DR. C. M. DOUGHERTY, Baton Rouge, Louisiana. This paper focuses attention on the effects of birth control pills upon a target tissue, the endometrial stroma. Previous studies have indicated a peculiar type of atrophy of endometrial glands brought on by combination type dosage schedules of administration. The production of adenomatous hyperplasia of the endocervix is a fairly well known phenomenon at this time. Papanicolaou smears show that there is probably an increase in squamous atypia in the cervices of pill users. In the finding of these histologic changes there has been agreement among several investigators, the agreement of findings tending to substantiate the conclusions.

Dr. Han has found evidence, in the endometrial stroma, of proliferated smooth muscle cells ("myometrial hyperplasia"). This observation of stimulation of smooth muscle is not entirely new, as the process has been reported in medical writings.

The discovery of two "early" endometrial stromal sarcoma growths in this series of 105 case studies was completely unexpected, and as far as I know unreported. Knowledge of additional facts, including the state of these two endometria before treatment with birth control pills, would be required before ascribing a cause-and-effect relationship in these cases. However, inasmuch as there are proliferative changes in other genital tract tissues the possibility should be considered. Even though the finding of stromal sarcoma was coincidental in these cases it would again emphasize the necessity for curettage of the uterus in instances of irregularity and abnormality of uterine bleeding.

Maqueo and associates[1] studied 317 women and found the only difference from normal endometrial histology was stromal edema in some treated endometria. He found no change in the endometrial or cytologic picture after several years of treatment.

Ober and associates[2] performed endometrial biopsies on 39 women treated with mestranol chlormadinone combination and cyclic dosage. No abnormal proliferative lesions were found.

Dr. Song made reference to two basic features of the endometrial stroma in supporting his hypothesis for explaining his observations. These are the embryonic origin of the endometrial stroma and the possibility of pluripotency of the stromal cell. It should be noted that the endometrial stroma is probably a development of the mesenchyme of the transverse septum of the pelvis in the early embryo. In the development of the Müllerian duct in these specimens there exists no definite organization of a ductal wall, but only a single-layered epithelial tube. Within the pelvis (about 30 mm. embryo) the epithelial tube is supported by mesenchymal tissue, which slowly condenses into myometrium, cervix, and myosalpinx. Whether the subepithelial stroma is formed from the mesenchyme or from proliferations of the Müllerian ductal epithelium is still not certain knowledge. There seem to be proponents of both modes of development.

The best evidence that the endometrial stroma is multipotent is its reputed capability to generate the mixed mesodermal tumor of the uterus, a tumor having muscle, bone, cartilage, and other nonuterine components. Suffice it to say we don't know quite as much about this process as we would like. Production of endometrial glands from endometrial stroma has been thought possible by some histologists. But when I asked one of my learned friends who was a morphologist (with a Ph.D. in histology) whether the one adult tissue could arise from the other, he gave me a frown of the type usually reserved for heretics. He simply couldn't admit the possibility of a gland cell originating from a connective tissue cell.

Whether or not these basic considerations are true or false, however, we might note that here is one more potential calamity to be on the lookout for among the patients taking The Pill.

REFERENCES
1. Maqueo, M., Bacerra, C., Munguia, H., and Goldzieher, J.: Amer. J. Obstet. Gynec. 90: 395, 1964.
2. Ober, William P., Decker, A., Clyman, M. J., and Roland, M.: Obstet. Gynec. 28: 247, 1966.

Dr. Alfred L. Kennan, Madison, Wisconsin. The Committee on Obstetrics and Gynecology of the Food and Drug Administration has just reviewed the "pills," and their report is under date of Aug. 1, 1969. This report is available now. One of the interesting things that appeared in this report was a description of 20 autopsies that had been done at the Armed Forces Institute of Pathology on young women who had apparently died of pulmonary embolus from the pill. In this report, the lesion that was considered characteristic was endothelial proliferation in small blood vessels. This was apparent in the lung vessels and in the vessels of the legs and other areas of the body. I think, for anyone who is interested in the unwanted effects of the pill, this report would be worthwhile reading.

Dr. Song (Closing). I believe we have gone as far as we could to describe the endometrial changes observed in women receiving oral contraceptives, as the morphology alone is rather limited and purely suggestive. We feel that we should reproduce those described changes experimentally, employing a sufficient number of monkeys and rabbits to confirm our observation. I do hope that we will be able to pursue this further experimentally.

111

Effect of oral contraceptives on human endometrium in culture

TIIU CSERMELY, Ph.D.

EDWARD C. HUGHES, M.D.

LAURENCE M. DEMERS, Ph.D.*

MANY INVESTIGATORS have described the histologic changes taking place in the human endometrium during cyclic administration of synthetic progestogen-estrogen combinations in oral contraceptive pills. In general, the combination type of pills cause premature secretory changes in the endometrial glands, followed by glandular regression and atrophy without fully developed secretion of the gland contents into the lumen. The endometrial stroma has a decidua-like appearance and the venules are often dilated.[6, 7, 12, 16]

The sequential pills produce a more normal type of endometrium. There is marked proliferation of both glands and stroma during the first part of the cycle when estrogen alone is administered. This is followed by a rapid secretory response under the influence

This work was supported by the Department of Health of the State of New York through the Empire State Medical, Scientific and Educational Foundation, Inc.

of the combination tablets during the second part of the cycle. There is no evidence of atrophy of either the glands or the stroma. Both the spiral arterioles and venules are minimally developed, and only a mild decidual reaction occurs. Several reports have indicated that the sequential regimen results in a delay of approximately 5 days in the development of secretory changes in the human endometrium as compared to the normal cycle.[6-8, 10, 11, 13, 14]

Blaustein, Shenker, and Post[1, 2] have recently reported that oral contraceptives, combination as well as sequential types, cause endothelial hyperplasia in sinusoids and spiral arterioles of the endometrium, as well as causing smooth muscle hyperplasia in the arteries. The latter has also been reported by Song, Mark, and Lawler.[16]

The nature of the endometrial response to oral contraceptives depends, at least partially, on the ovulatory and hormonal status of the women taking these drugs.[15] Therefore, one can only speculate as to whether the endometrial changes are caused by a direct action of the synthetic hormones on the endometrium, or whether these effects are secondary to disturbances in the hor-

Table I. Oral contraceptives used in this investigation

Brand name	Estrogen component	Progesterone component	No. of specimens
Ortho-Novum 2 mg.	Mestranol, 0.10 mg.	Norethindrone, 2 mg.	8
Ortho-Novum 1/80	Mestranol, 0.08 mg.	Norethindrone, 1 mg.	7
Ortho-Novum SQ, blue	Mestranol, 0.08 mg.	Norethindrone, 2 mg.	9
Ortho-Novum SQ, white	Mestranol, 0.08 mg.	—	8
Norinyl 1 + 80	Mestranol, 0.08 mg.	Norethindrone, 1 mg.	9
Ovulen	Mestranol, 0.10 mg.	Ethynodiol diacetate, 1 mg.	12
Provest	Ethinyl estradiol, 0.05 mg.	Medroxyprogesterone acetate, 10 mg.	22
Ovral	Ethinyl estradiol, 0.05 mg.	Norgestrel, 0.5 mg.	9
Enovid E	Mestranol, 0.10 mg.	Norethynodrel, 2.5 mg.	11
C-Quens	Mestranol, 0.08 mg.	Chlormadinone acetate, 2 mg.	11

monal pattern exerted at the level of the hypothalamic-pituitary-ovarian axis.

We have previously shown that human endometrium, removed from the influences and interactions of other organs in in vitro cultures, responds in a fairly predictable and physiologic way to added progesterone or estradiol.[4, 5, 9] We have now extended these studies to investigate the direct effects of oral contraceptives on human endometrial cultures in vitro, using the results obtained with the natural ovarian steroids as a basis for comparison.

Material and methods

A total of 82 specimens of human endometrium, obtained by curettage and taken during different parts of the menstrual cycle, were used in this investigation. Normal patients as well as women with problems of infertility or dysfunctional bleeding were included in this group. A portion of each specimen was used for initial histologic and biochemical evaluation to provide a base line for comparisons. Tissue glycogen content was determined using a phenol mixture as described by Montgomery. Standard histologic and histochemical methods were used. After fixation in absolute alcohol the tissue was embedded in paraffin and sectioned at a thickness of 6 μ. The slides were stained with hen. atoxylin and eosin, periodic acid–Schiff reagent (P.A.S.) for glycogen, and a modified Gomori stain for alkaline phosphatase activity. The same methods were used to evaulate the tissue explants after varying periods of time in organ culture.

The culture method used in this work, a modification of the one described by Trowell, was the same as for our previous studies.[4] Small pieces of human endometrium, cut to a size of about 2 mm.[3], were placed on Gelman Metricel filters in Falcon polystyrene organ culture dishes. Each dish held 5 endometrial explants and about 1 ml. of culture medium (Trowell's T8 medium containing 10 per cent fetal calf serum, 100 units of penicillin, 100 μg of streptomycin, and 0.25 μg of Fungizone per milliliter; Grand Island Biological Company). The culture dishes were incubated for a period of 1 to 4 days in an atmosphere of 95 per cent O_2 and 5 per cent CO_2 at 37° C. At the end of the incubation period two of the explants were immediately fixed for histologic and histochemical evaluation, and the remaining three were analyzed for glycogen content.

The oral contraceptives studied and the number of specimens on which each one was tested are listed in Table I. Each tablet was suspended in 10 ml. of water and an aliquot of this suspension was added to the culture medium to give the desired concentration which was 1/1,000 of a tablet per milliliter unless specified otherwise. In a number of cases the concentrations were varied to include both 1/2,000 tablet per milliliter and 1/500 tablet per milliliter. At these concentrations there was no apparent precipitation and all the ingredients were assumed to be in solution.

Control cultures containing the same medium but without added ho.:nones were set up from every specimen and maintained

113

Table II. Glycogen content of endometrial explants

Specimen No.	Patient status	Day of cycle	Days in culture	Glycogen content with given supplement*								
				None	Ortho-Novum SQ,white	Ortho-Novum 1/80	Ortho-Novum 2 mg.	Pro-vest	Ovral	C-Quens	Enovid E	Progesterone 0.5 µg/ml.
89	Bleeder	13	0	184								
			2	172	121			600	407			
100	Bleeder	15	0	272								
			1	579	474		790	938	735			
			4	126	100		538	220	359			
131	Normal	19	0	480								
			2	405				607	791			766
144	Normal	17	0	580								
			2	299					1632			
154	Normal	12	0	262								
			2	92		640		571				862
265	Aborter	20	0	trace								
			2	194						427	746	
270	Aborter	18	0	212								
			3	277						500		

*Glycogen is expressed as milligrams per 100 mg. of tissue (wet weight). Concentration of contraceptives 1/1,000 tablets per milliliter of medium.

along with the experimental cultures. In some cases estradiol- or progesterone-supplemented cultures were also evaluated for purposes of comparison.

Since the contraceptive pills rather than the chemically pure steroids were used in this study, it was necessary to demonstrate that the carbohydrate vehicle of the pills did not affect the endometrial explants. To do this, we tested two kinds of the placebo pills (Norinyl 1 + 80, pink tablet, and Ovulen, pink tablet) in a manner identical to tests with pills containing active ingredients.

In addition to the specimens to which synthetic steroids were added in vitro, we also obtained biopsy specimens from 10 normal women who were taking oral contraceptives, so that the results from cultured specimens could be compared to the in vivo response of the tissue.

Results

The effects of incubation in vitro, as shown by the control cultures, were the same as in our previous studies.[4, 5, 9] There was variable central necrosis with time, the stroma often became a little more compact,

the glands increased slightly in size, and there was a tendency toward stratification of epithelial cell nuclei. The tissue glycogen content decreased gradually with time, as shown both biochemically and histochemically.

The results from the experiments with inert tablets were similar to the ones of control cultures. There were no noticeable histologic or histochemical effects, and no changes in the glycogen levels as compared to the control cultures.

The preparation containing only mestranol (Ortho-Novum SQ, white tablet) produced changes in the endometrial explants similar to those caused by supplementation of the culture medium with estradiol. There was considerable stratification of the epithelial cell nuclei, some variation in size of glands, appearance of occasional cystic glands, increased stromal density, and prominence of blood vessels. In some specimens mestranol supplementation caused alterations in the pattern of stromal cells. The cells tended to be arranged in swirls, especially around glands and around blood vessels. The glycogen content of the explants tended to be a

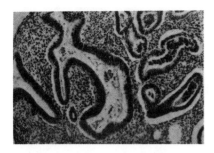

Fig. 1. Specimen No. 139, taken on Day 16 of the cycle, cultured for 2 days in medium containing Ortho-Novum SQ, white tablet (mestranol). (Hematoxylin and eosin. ×100.)

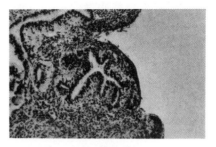

Fig. 2. Same specimen as in Fig. 1, cultured for 2 days in medium containing Ortho-Novum 2 mg. (mestranol and norethindrone). Note subnuclear vacuoles and secretory nature of glands. (Hematoxylin and eosin. ×100.)

little lower than in the control cultures (Table II). There was no mestranol-induced change in the histochemically detectable alkaline phosphatase activity.

The histologic appearance of a specimen cultured for 2 days in mestranol-supplemented medium is shown in Fig. 1. For comparison, Fig. 2 shows the same specimen after 2 days in medium containing Ortho-Novum 2 mg.

The proliferative changes due to mestranol were more noticeable than those caused by addition of estradiol and could be seen even in a specimen obtained on Day 29 of the cycle. Neither 0.5 μg of estradiol per milliliter nor 0.5 μg of progesterone per milliliter had any appreciable histologic effect on this specimen after 2 days in organ culture. Mestranol, in a concentration of 0.04 μg per milliliter (1/2,000 Ortho-Novum SQ white tablet per milliliter), also failed to have any effect, but in concentrations of 0.08 μg per milliliter and 0.16 μg per milliliter it caused increased stratification in the glands. In addition, these amounts of mestranol also produced histochemically detectable glycogen deposits in the walls of the blood vessels.

All of the progestogen-estrogen containing preparations produced secretory changes in the endometrial explants which resembled those produced by supplementation with a combination of estradiol and progesterone. However, in addition to the increased size of the glands, increased stratification, develop-

ment of subnuclear vacuoles, and increased deposition of glycogen in these vacuoles, there were some additional changes in the tissue which seemed to be characteristic of oral contraceptives and were not observed with estradiol-progesterone combinations. These included a tendency of stromal cells to form swirling patterns around the glands and blood vessels, formation of glycogen-containing vacuoles at the tips of glandular epithelial cells in addition to the subnuclear ones, increased glycogen in the stroma, and thickening of the walls of the blood vessels. The nuclei of the glandular epithelial cells tended to be large and round. The stromal cells were often round and decidua-like, containing glycogen, although stromal density varied from very compact to loose.

Figs. 3 and 5 show the appearance of two of the specimens after 2 days incubation in the control medium, while Figs. 4 and 6 show explants from the same specimens after the same period of incubation in media containing contraceptive tablets. Prominent secretory vacuoles were produced by the contraceptives in both specimens, although one was obtained during the early part of the menstrual cycle and the other during the secretory phase.

Tissue glycogen levels, as determined both histochemically and by biochemical analysis, were increased not only when compared to the control cultures but also when compared to the initial glycogen levels of the speci-

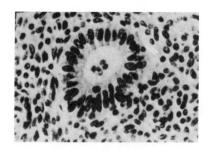

Fig. 3. Specimen No. 264, taken on Day 4 of the cycle, cultured for 2 days in control medium. (Hematoxylin and eosin. ×540.)

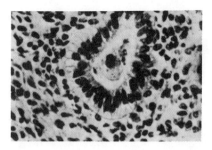

Fig. 4. Same specimen as in Fig. 3, cultured for 2 days in medium containing C-Quens. Note subnuclear vacuoles. (Hematoxylin and eosin. ×540.)

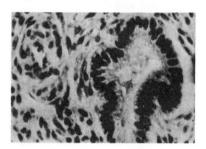

Fig. 5. Specimen No. 131, taken on Day 20 of the cycle, cultured for 2 days in control medium. Note secretory nature of gland. (Hematoxylin and eosin. ×540.)

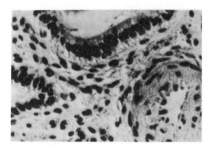

Fig. 6. Same specimen as in Fig. 5, cultured for 2 days in medium containing Ovral. Note subnuclear vacuoles, concentric pattern of stromal cells around gland, and thick-walled blood vessel. (Hematoxylin and eosin. ×540.)

mens. The glycogen levels of a number of typical specimens are given in Table II. On P.A.S. stained slides the glycogen could be seen in huge globules, often both at the base and at the luminal edges of the epithelial cells, some globules being released into the gland lumen. Stromal cells were especially rich in glycogen in the immediate vicinity of the glands. In a number of specimens there was glycogen in the walls of the blood vessels.

The alkaline phosphatase activity was increased in all the synthetic progestogen-treated specimens, being located mostly in the upper half of the epithelial cells, in their nuclei and in the lumen.

All of the contraceptives tested, as well as natural progesterone and estradiol, produced their maximal effects in approximately 2 days in organ culture. The first histologically detectable changes appeared after 18 to 20 hours, and by 24 hours biochemically determined glycogen was considerably increased.

No dose-related differences were noted when the concentrations of Ortho-Novum SQ (blue tablet), Ortho-Novum 1/80, Provest, Ovral, or Ovulen were varied. Concentrations of 1/2,000 tablet per milliliter, 1/1,000 tablet per milliliter, and 1/500 tablet per milliliter resulted in the same typical response, both histologically and biochemically, suggesting a wide range of doses where an "all or none" relationship exists.

Regardless of some variation from specimen to specimen, the endometrial response

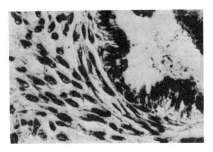

Fig. 7. Specimen obtained on Day 7 of the cycle from patient on Ortho-Novum 1/80. Note crowding of epithelial cell nuclei and concentric pattern of stromal cells around gland. (Hematoxylin and eosin. ×540.)

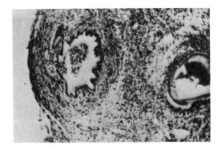

Fig. 8. Specimen obtained on Day 19 of the cycle from patient on Ovulen. Note cystic gland and arrangement of stromal cells around glands (Periodic acid–Schiff stain. ×540.)

to the contraceptive agents did not seem to vary greatly with the phase of the cycle, the clinical condition of the women, or with the specific preparation used. An exception to this were some specimens where Provest as well as Ovral were tested, and the histologic secretory response was more pronounced with Provest, although the tissue glycogen levels were comparably increased with both.

The differences in the mestranol/norethindrone ratio in the three different Ortho-Novum preparations (0.10 mg. per 2 mg., 0.08 mg. per 1 mg. and 0.08 mg. per 2 mg.) did not affect either the histologic or biochemical results obtained. A typical response was obtained with any of these tablets, including proliferative as well as secretory changes in the tissue.

Both the oral contraceptives containing the 17-hydroxyprogesterone derivatives (norethindrone, ethynodiol diacetate, norgestrel, norethynodrel) and the ones with the 19-nortestosterone derivatives (medroxyprogesterone acetate, chlormadinone acetate) had a similar effect on the endometrial explants.

Nine of the 10 women who were taking oral contraceptives were on the combination type pills (Ovulen, Ortho-Novum 2 mg., Ortho-Novum 1 mg., Ortho-Novum 1/80, Enovid, and Oracon). Of these, 2 had had amenorrhea of several months' duration at the time of biopsy, and for the rest the day of cycle at the time of biopsy ranged from 7 to 26. In addition to the expected secretory

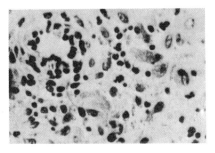

Fig. 9. Specimen obtained from a patient after long-term Enovid therapy. Note extreme decidual reaction. (Hematoxylin and eosin. ×540.)

changes, there were considerable amounts of glycogen in the stromal cells in all of these specimens. This glycogen was heaviest around the glands and blood vessels, and appeared to be granular in nature. Five of the specimens also showed swirling patterns of stromal cells and one had glycogen in the walls of blood vessels. The histologic appearance of two of these specimens is shown in Figs. 7 and 8. The single specimen from a woman taking the sequential type of pills (Ortho-Novum SQ) was obtained on Day 10 of the cycle, and showed, in addition to proliferative changes, also a small amount of glycogen in the stroma and in the walls of the blood vessels.

Fig. 9 shows endometrium from a patient after long-term Enovid therapy, and demonstrates an extreme decidual reaction.

117

Comment

Although the oral contraceptives are in wide general use, their exact mode of action is not fully understood. In addition to inhibiting ovulation, the synthetic steroids may have effects on fertilization and transport of ova in the Fallopian tubes, on implantation, on physicochemical properties of cervical mucus, and on the endometrium.[6]

The results of this investigation show that isolated human endometrial explants respond to the synthetic estrogens and progestogens in oral contraceptives, and that the response is in many respects similar to the response of the same tissue to natural ovarian steroids. However, there are several differences which are, as yet, unexplained, and which were also found when the contraceptives were administered to the patients. The most obvious of these are the deposition of considerable amounts of glycogen in the stromal cells, and the swirling patterns of stromal cells around the glands. The latter has also been mentioned by Cittadini, Quartararo, and Romano[3] who described it as fused-like cells around the glands. In our experience neither of these findings was limited to any one contraceptive or any type of chemical component of the pills, and both appear to be characteristic effects of oral contraceptives.

Summary

Specimens of human endometrium were maintained in vitro in media supplemented with a number of oral contraceptives in order to determine the direct effect of these compounds on the endometrium. The effects were evaluated histologically, histochemically, and biochemically. All of the contraceptives tested affected the tissue in a manner similar to their effects in vivo. Mestranol caused proliferative changes, while progestogens induced secretory changes, elevated tissue glycogen levels, and glycogen deposition in the stromal cells as well as in sub- and supranuclear vacuoles in the epithelial cells. All of the contraceptives were responsible for prominence of blood vessels and for characteristic swirling patterns of stromal cells around the glands and blood vessels.

REFERENCES

1. Blaustein, A., and Shenker, L.: Obstet. Gynec. 35: 12, 1970.
2. Blaustein, A., Shenker, L., and Post, R. C.: Int. J. Fertil. 13: 466, 1968.
3. Cittadini, E., Quartararo, P., and Romano, F.: Int. J. Fertil. 14: 180, 1969.
4. Csermely, T., Demers, L. M., and Hughes, E. C.: Obstet. Gynec. 34: 252, 1969.
5. Demers, L. M., Csermely, T., and Hughes, E. C.: Obstet. Gynec. 36: 275, 1970.
6. Diczfalusy, E.: AMER. J. OBSTET. GYNEC. 100: 136, 1968.
7. Friedrich, E. R.: Obstet. Gynec. 30: 201, 1967.
8. Goldzieher, J. W., Becerra, C., Gual, C., Livingston, N. B., Maqueo, M., Moses, L. E., and Tietze, C.: AMER. J. OBSTET. GYNEC. 90: 404, 1964.
9. Hughes, E. C., Demers, L. M., Csermely, T., and Jones, D. B.: AMER. J. OBSTET. GYNEC. 105: 707, 1969.
10. Hutcherson, W. P., Schwartz, H. A., Weathers, W., and McGuire, J. E.: Fertil. Steril. 18: 616, 1967.
11. Maqueo, M., Becerra, C., Munguia, H., and Goldzieher, J. W.: AMER. J. OBSTET. GYNEC. 90: 395, 1964.
12. Maqueo, M., Perez-Vega, E., Goldzieher, J. W., Martinez-Manautou, J., and Rudel, H.: AMER. J. OBSTET. GYNEC. 85: 427, 1963.
13. Ober, W. B., Decker, A., Clyman, M. J., and Roland, M.: Obstet. Gynec. 28: 247, 1966.
14. Parkinson, R. W., McQuarrie, H. G., Ellsworth, H. S., and Stone, R. A.: Obstet. Gynec. 28: 239, 1966.
15. Roland, M., Clyman, M. J., Decker, A., and Ober, W. B.: Fertil. Steril. 15: 143, 1964.
16. Song, J., Mark, M. S., and Lawler, M. P.: AMER. J. OBSTET. GYNEC. 107: 717, 1970.

ALKALINE PHOSPHATASE CONCENTRATION IN CERVICAL MUCUS*

D. C. SMITH, W. B. HUNTER, and L. R. SPADONI

Since the introduction of a histochemical technic for demonstrating alkaline phosphatase in tissues by Gomori[7] in 1939, numerous reports have appeared in the literature related to the activity of this enzyme in many of the tissues of the female genital tract, including the endometrium and endocervical and vaginal mucosa.[9, 12, 19] Of particular interest has been the activity present in the cytoplasm of the endometrial and endocervical epithelium, which has been shown to exhibit cyclic changes corresponding to the menstrual cycle, with increasing amounts of enzymatic activity seen during the proliferative phase of the cycle followed by gradual diminishing of enzyme activity during the secretory phase. On the other hand, the endocervical mucosa of postmenopausal women has been shown to exhibit very little alkaline phosphatase activity. This can be reversed by the administration of estrogen.[9] Additional evidence of the apparent response of alkaline phosphatase to estrogenic stimulation has been the increased activity of this enzyme in the granular leukocytes of peripheral blood during normal menstrual cycles and with the administered estrogen. Quantification of the leukocyte alkaline phosphatase activity has been advocated in the past as an early test for pregnancy.[8]

Because of the response of the endometrial and endocervical mucosa to estrogen stimulation, a study was undertaken to measure the alkaline phosphatase activ-

* This study was supported by National Institute of Health Grant T1 AM 05428-06, and was presented in part at the Pacific Coast Fertility Society's 16th Annual Meeting, Palm Springs, California, November 1968.

ity of the cervical mucus to define its response to hormonal stimulus.

METHODS

Patients included in the study were divided into three categories.

1. Normal women of reproductive age, with regular ovulatory cycles, not using any method of contraception were selected. Serial cervical mucus specimens were obtained beginning on approximately the 10th day of the cycle and continuing until the mucus could no longer be obtained following the ovulatory period. Evidence of ovulation was determined using conventional parameters, including basal body temperature and the character and amount of the cervical mucus.

2. Patients in the second category were receiving gonadotropin therapy (human menopausal gonadotrophin (Cutter Laboratories, Berkeley, Calif.) human chorionic gonadotrophin (Ayerst Laboratories, New York, N. Y.)). Patients in this group were being treated with gonadotropins for anovulation and infertility. Parameters used to follow ovarian response were urinary estriol excretion rates, ovarian size, and cervical mucus, as well as the shift of basal body temperature as an index of ovulation.

3. Patients in this group were given a variety of estrogen and progestational drugs in sequence and combination. In this category, several different estrogenic and progestational drugs were administered to patients to determine their effect on cervical mucus alkaline phosphatase. In several patients 24-hr. urine collections were obtained simultaneously and the

estriol content was measured as an indication of estrogen secretion.[23]

The cervical mucus specimens were obtained in serial fashion during the normal menstrual or treatment cycles in the following manner. The cervix was wiped clean with a cotton swab and the cervical

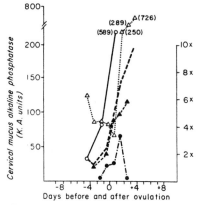

Fig. 1. Changes in cervical mucus alkaline phosphatase in normal ovulating women. (The *heavy interrupted line* represents the average relative change of all of the individual curves.)

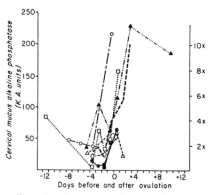

Fig. 2. Serial mucus alkaline phosphatase values in patients receiving human menopausal gonadotropin-human chorionic gonadotropin therapy. (The *heavy interrupted line* represents the average relative change of all of the individual curves.)

mucus was aspirated with a 1-cc. tuberculin syringe. After transfer to a clean test tube, the mucus was digested by the addition of approximately 0.5 mg. of trypsin (Worthington Biochemical Corporation, Freehold, N. J.). The amount of alkaline phosphatase activity was then determined in an aliquot of 0.02 ml. by a modification of the method described by Kaplan and Narahara[11] (0.2 ml. of mucus added to 3 ml. of substrate buffered with 0.1 M Na_2CO_3). The results are expressed in King-Armstrong units.

RESULTS

Normal Ovulatory Cycles. The values in 4 patients with regular cycles are seen in Fig 1. Preovulatory levels of mucus alkaline phosphatase showed a wide variation among individual patients but showed no significant elevation until the day after ovulation, when there was a marked upward trend in enzymatic activity. At this time and during the ensuing several days, high values of alkaline phosphatase activity were obtained and, except for one determination, persisted as long as mucus was available for measurement.

Patients Receiving Human Menopausal Gonadotropin-Human Chorionic Gonadotropin Therapy. Variations were observed in the preovulatory or base line phase; however, each patient exhibited a marked rise in mucus phosphatase activity within 24 hr of the time of presumptive ovulation (Fig. 2). Because of the impossibility of determining the exact time of ovulation by conventional means, an accurate correlation of this phenomenon and phosphatase rise was not possible. However, it appeared that a significant increase in phosphatase activity occurred in the mucus of these patients on the day prior to basal body temperature elevation and continued in an upward fashion to a peak some 2.3 days following ovulation. Estriol excretion measurements obtained at the same time as cervical mucus specimens showed no correlation between total estriol output and mucus phosphatase activity.

Patients Treated with Estrogen-Progestagen Combination Oral Contraception. Five patients were studied while taking a sequential oral contraceptive, C-Quens Lilly and Co., Indianapolis, Ind.), containing mestranol (17α-ethynyl estradiol-3-methyl ether) (80 mcg. for 15 days), and 5 days of combination mestranol (80 mcg.) and chlormadinone acetate (6-chloro-Δ6-dehydro-17α-acetoxyprogesterone) ; 2-mg. serial cervical mucus specimens were obtained during both the phase of mestranol administration alone and during the phase of combined therapy with mestranol and chlormadinone. As seen in Fig. 3, rather consistent levels of alkaline phosphatase activity are observed during the first 15 days (mestranol only), although there is some variation in base line levels among the individual patients. However, 48 hr. after the administration of chlormadinone there was a marked increase in phosphatase activity. This pattern of alkaline phosphatase rise with a progestogen could be duplicated by administering mestranol for 15 days followed by mestranol in combination with norethindrone (17α-ethynyl-19-nortestosterone), 2 mg. (Ortho-Novum, Ortho Pharmaceuticals, Raritan, N. J.) (Fig. 4). Similar magnitudes of phosphatase elevation were seen in 2 patients treated with this regimen. Estriol excretion patterns obtained in patients taking sequential oral contraception were extremely low, because of pituitary and ovarian suppression by the medication, with values ranging from undetectable amounts to usually less than 5 mcg./24 hr.

Two additional patients were treated in a similar sequential fashion using Premarin, Ayerst Laboratories, New York, N. Y. (conjugated equine estrogens), 5 mg. daily for 15 days, and Provera Upjohn Company, Kalamazoo, Mich. (17α hydroxy-6α-methyl progesterone), 10 mg. daily in combination for 5 days. Again a

marked elevation of the concentration of alkaline phosphatase in the mucus was observed 48 hr. after the progestational agent had been administered (Fig. 5). In contrast to the low estriol excretion patterns ex-

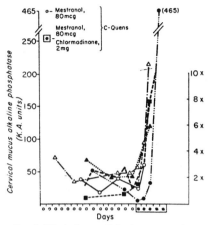

Fig. 3. Effect of sequential estrogen-progestagen administration on cervical mucus alkaline phosphatase concentration. (The *heavy interrupted line* represents the average relative change of all of the individual curves.)

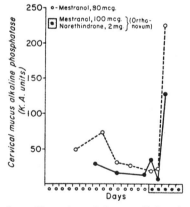

Fig. 4. Change in cervical mucus alkaline phosphatase concentration by the administration of a 19 nor-testosterone compound to patients receiving daily estrogen.

121

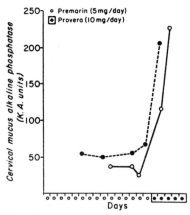

FIG. 5. Change in cervical mucus alkaline phosphatase concentration by the administration of Provera (17 hydroxy-6-methyl progesterone) to patients receiving daily estrogen.

hibited by the patients taking the synthetic estrogens, much higher estriol levels were observed in the 2 patients, ranging from 20–60 mcg./24 hr., probably representing the excretion product of the administered conjugated estrogens. There was no observable difference in base line phosphatase values, in spite of the elevated estriol excretion.

Direct evidence of the effect of progesterone was seen following the administration of 25 mg. of aqueous progesterone (Fig. 6) intramuscularly to 2 patients who were treated with 80 gm. of mestranol daily. Marked elevations in the phosphatase activity were observed within 48 hr. after the injection of progesterone. This was succeeded by a return to base line or near base line levels after 5 days. At this time, chlormadinone acetate, 2 mg., was administered and again this was accompanied by a significant rise in the mucus alkaline phosphatase activity. The latter experiment was carried out to determine whether a previous marked rise in phosphatase would tend to deplete the mucus enzyme activity and prevent a subsequent

increase when another progestational agent was administered.

Other hormones tested for their effect on mucus alkaline phosphatase were Duphasten (Phillips Roxanne Laboratories, Columbus, Ohio) (6-dehydro-9β,10α-progesterone), which also was accompanied by a rise in enzyme concentration, and human chorionic gonadotropin, which had no effect.

DISCUSSION

Phosphatases in general belong to a group of enzymes that possess the ability to split phosphate or phosphoric acid from various phosphate esters. The alkaline phosphatases which we are concerned with are phosphomonoesterases, i.e., capable of hydrolyzing monoesters of orthophosphoric acid. The technic used to quantitate the enzyme in cervical mucus, when used on serum, may well provide a measurement of

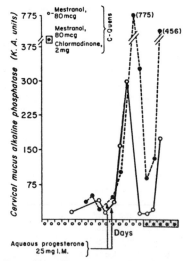

FIG. 6. The effect of a single injection of aqueous progesterone on cervical mucus alkaline phosphatase. After the return of mucus phosphatase values to near base line levels, the subsequent administration of a second progestational agent results in another increase in enzyme activity.

the sum of several different alkaline phosphatases and not a specific enzyme.[10] Recent advances in technics, including agar gel electrophoresis[26] and gel filtration,[5] have enabled differentiation of tissue of origin; however, these procedures were not employed in the present study. It is assumed that the enzyme activity measured in the mucus reflects secretions from the endometrial and endocervical mucosa.

Alkaline phosphatase activity in the endometrium and endocervical mucosa has been studied rather extensively and generally shows a cyclic variation with the menstrual cycle with increasing amounts of enzyme activity occurring during the proliferative phase or with exogenous estrogen administration and diminishing amounts after ovulation. Similar observations have been made in normal and ovariectomized monkeys when treated with exogenous estrogens.[1, 18] When progesterone was combined with estrogen, there was a marked reduction in the epithelial alkaline phosphatase, with a shift to the luminal secretions.

Although alkaline phosphatase has been found to be significantly higher in menstrual discharge sera than in the bloodstream, there are few reports to be found in the literature regarding alkaline phosphatase in the cervical mucus. High levels of alkaline phosphatase were found in the vaginal mucus of heifers just prior to estrus,[24] and there are two reports of phosphatase activity in human cervical mucus at a comparable time in the cycle, allegedly produced in response to estrogen.[6] This was not substantiated by the present study, where the findings seem to indicate increases in enzyme activity due to progestational stimulation.

The reasons for this discrepancy remain obscure; however, the effect of the thickening or concentration of the cervical mucus under the influence of progesterone might contribute to this observation. No attempt was made to correlate enzyme activity with mucus volume or dry weight of mucus; however, the marked increase observed in many patients from one day to the next would not seem to be accounted for as a result of increased mucus concentration alone. The contribution of alkaline phosphatase from leukocytes appearing in the mucus after ovulation must also be considered and investigated further. Mc-Kay et al.[19] described alkaline phosphatase activity in the endometrial epithelial cells which appeared in the luminal tips in increasing amounts during the proliferative phase, peaking at midcycle.

During the early secretory phase, the activity in the glandular cell tips gradually decreased in amount until Day 22, when it was no longer seen in the cytoplasm and a shift in location to the secretion within the glandular lumina was noted. This decrease in epithelial cytoplasm and the appearance of the enzyme in the lumina of the glands roughly coincides with the relatively high levels of alkaline phosphatase in the mucus presenting at the cervical os, and perhaps may be an explanation for the marked increase in enzyme activity at this time. It is evident that there is no significant change in the mucus alkaline phosphatase during the follicular phase of the cycle or with the administration of exogeneous estrogens, and that the rise is seen only at or after ovulation or with the administration of various progestational compounds. Other investigators have suggested that increases in leukocyte alkaline phosphatase activity might also be due to progesterone stimulation.[3, 20]

Whether or not the presence of alkaline phosphatase in high concentration in the cervical mucus is significant from a physiologic standpoint or merely a reflection of secretion or desquamation of cytoplasmic contents of metabolically active epithelial cells is a matter of speculation. Previous work by McLeod[15, 16] has stressed the importance of glycolytic energy pathways in sperm metabolism and motility, and numerous papers have appeared describing carbohydrates present in cervical mucus.[2, 13, 23, 25] Increased reduction of these mucus sugars by the addition of spermatozoa has been shown by Lipphart,[14] and the possible participation of alkaline phosphatases and other enzymes in this scheme of carbohydrate utilization becomes an interesting but, as yet, unanswered question.

REFERENCES

1. ATKINSON, W. B., AND ENGLE, E. T. Studies on endometrial alkaline phosphatase during the human menstrual cycle and in the hormone treated monkey. Endocrinology 40:327, 1947.
2. BERGMAN, P., AND WERNER, I. Analysis of carbohydrates in human cervical mucus by means of paper partition chromatography.
3. CLIMIE, A. R. W., HEINRICHS, W. L., AND FOSTER, I. J. Neutrophilic alkaline phosphatase test. Amer J Clin Path 38:95, 1962.
4. DeMERRE, L. J., AND LITOFSKY, F. S. Alkaline phosphatase activity during menstruation. Fertil Steril 19:593, 1968.
5. DUNNE, J., FENNELLY, S. J., AND McGEENEY, K. Separation of alkaline phosphatase enzymes in human serum using gel filtration (Sephadex G-200). Techniques Cancer 20:71, 1967.
6. GIBBONS, R. A., AND MATTNER, P. Some aspects of the chemistry of cervical mucus. Int J Fertil 11:366, 1966.
7. GOMORI, G. Microtechnical demonstration of phosphatase in tissue sections. Proc Soc Exp Biol Med 42:23, 1939.
8. HARER, W. B., JR., AND QUIGLEY, H. J. Alkaline

9. HEDBERG, G. T. The alkaline phosphatase activity in the cervical mucosa. Gynaecologia (Basel) 128:239, 1950.
10. HENRY. R. J. Clinical Chemistry Principles and Techniques, Hoeber, Harper and Row, New York, 1965, 484.
11. KAPLAN, A., AND NASCHARA, A. J. Lab-Clin Med 41:814, 1953.
12. LANG, W. R., RAKOFF, A. E., AND GRESS, M. Alkaline phosphatase in vaginal biopsies. Amer J Obstet Gynec 68:815, 1954.
13. LAPAN, X. X., AND FRIEDMAN, M. M. Glycopus and reducing substances in vaginal mucus. Amer J Obst and Gynec 59:921, 1950.
14. LIPPHARDT, E. M., AND POMMERENKE, W. T. Effect of addition of spermatozoa on the sugar content of cervical mucous. Amer J Obstet Gynec 59:918, 1950.
15. MacLEOD, J. The metabolism of human spermatozoa. Amer J Physiol 132:193, 1941.
16. MacLEOD, J. The effect of glycolysis inhibitors and of certain substrates on the metabolism and motility of human spermatozoa. Endocrinology 29:583, 1941.
17. MAHLER, H. R. AND CORDES, E. H. Biological Chemistry, Harper and Row, New York, 1900.
18. MANNING, J. P., HISOW. R. L., STEINETZ, B. G., AND KROC, R. L. The effects of ovarian hormones on uterine phosphatases of the rhesus monkey. Anat Rec 157:465, 1967.
19. McKAY, ET AL. Histochemical observations on the endometrium—normal. Obstet Gynec 8:22, 1956.
20. O'KELL, R. T., AND AXON, L. L. Leukocyte alkaline phosphatase in the newborn infant. Amer Obstet Gynec 93:1181, 1965.
21. POLISHUK, W. Z., ZUCKERMAN, H., AND DIAMANTE, Y. Alkaline phosphatase activity in leukocytes during menstrual cycle. Fertil Steril 19:901, 1968.
22. SCHINDLER, A. E., AND HERRMANN, W. L. Determination of steroids by gas liquid chromatography. Gynaecologia (Basel) 161:446, 1961.
23. SHETTLES, L. R. The polysaccharide composition of human cervical mucous. Fertil Steril 2:361, 1951.
24. VAN KLINKENBERG, G. A. Extremely high alkaline phosphatase activity in the vaginal mucous of the cow. Nature (London) 172:397, 1953.
25. VIERGIVER, E., AND POMMERENKE, W. T. The determination of reducing substances in human cervical mucus. Amer J Obstet Gynec 54:459, 1947.
26. YONG, J. M. Origins of serum alkaline phosphatase. J Clin Path 29:647, 1967.

phosphatase activity in granular leukocytes as a test for early pregnancy. Obstet Gynec 17: 238. 1961.

Effect of oral contraceptives on serum protein concentrations

HIRAM W. MENDENHALL, M.D.

THE EXTENSIVE metabolic alterations produced by high levels of circulating ovarian steroids are most clearly manifested in pregnancy. In addition to the changes in salt and water metabolism and the obvious morphologic changes in reproductive tract tissues accompanying heightened protein anabolism, alterations in the concentrations of several serum proteins have been documented.[1] Following administration of estrogens to nonpregnant individuals, changes in serum protein patterns similar to those observed in pregnant patients have been detected by several investigators.[2, 3] They also observed an increase in the concentration of some proteins, a decrease in the concentration of others, and no change in the level of many. In some instances the effect appears dependent upon both the dosage of steroid and the length of time of administration.[4] The significance and implications of these changes is poorly understood at present.

Use of oral contraceptives has been de-

scribed as producing a "metabolic pseudopregnancy."[5] In the present study, the effect of oral contraceptive usage on the concentrations of 8 serum proteins has been investigated. The values determined are contrasted with those seen in the pregnant patient at term.

Materials and methods

Eight separate proteins representative of the major electrophoretic fractions of serum have been measured by the technique of single radial immunodiffusion. Venous blood was drawn from 20 healthy women in the reproductive age group, at different stages in the menstrual cycle, who were receiving a variety of sequential and combination-type oral contraceptives including Ortho-Novum (norethindrone 2 mg. and mestranol 0.1 mg.), Enovid-E (norethynodrel 5 mg. and mestranol 0.075 mg.), Ovulen (ethynodiol diacetate 1 mg. and mestranol 0.1 mg.), Norinyl (norethindrone 2 mg. and mestranol 0.1 mg.), and Oracon (ethinyl estradiol 0.1 mg. alone or with 25 mg. dimethisterone) for periods ranging from 2 months to 7 years.

Antigens and antisera were prepared, and serum protein concentrations were measured as previously described.[1] The control group consisted of 25 healthy women in the reproductive age period. The levels of albumin,

This work was supported in part by the 1967 National Institutes of Health General Research Support Grant No. 5-501-FR-05362-07 at the University of Florida College of Medicine.

125

Table I. Serum protein concentrations (mean values ± 1 S.D.)

	Albumin (mg. %)	IgG (mg. %)	IgM (mg. %)	IgA (mg. %)	Cerulo-plasmin (%)	Trans-ferrin (%)	α_2-Macro-globulin (%)	α_1-Anti-trypsin (%)
Nonpregnant women	4,296 ± 451	1,248 ± 408	89 ± 28	241 ± 142	100	100	100	100
Oral con-traceptives	3,800 ± 463	1,165 ± 291	114 ± 46	201 ± 100	213 ± 61	120 ± 34	80 ± 17	244 ± 46
P values*	< 0.001	> 0.4	< 0.05	> 0.2				

*P = probability that the difference between means is due to chance (Student's t test of paired variables).

Table II. Comparison of serum protein concentrations in pregnancy (at term) and in women using oral contraceptives

	Albumin (mg. %)	IgG (mg. %)	IgM (mg. %)	IgA (mg. %)	Cerulo-plasmin (%)	Trans-ferrin (%)	α_2-Macro-globulin (%)	α_1-Anti-trypsin (%)
Pregnant women	3,144 ± 709	1,571 ± 598	123 ± 52	242 ± 146	234 ± 67	160 ± 49	110 ± 34	324 ± 90
Oral contra-ceptives	3,800 ± 463	1,165 ± 291	114 ± 46	201 ± 100	213 ± 61	120 ± 34	80 ± 17	244 ± 46

IgG, IgM, and IgA were measured in the serum of each of these women and for ceruloplasmin, transferrin, α_2-macroglobulin, and α_1-antitrypsin a pool of their sera was chosen as a normal reference serum.

Results

In Table I, the mean concentrations of the 8 proteins measured in the sera of women receiving oral contraceptives are contrasted with the values detected in the control sera. Whereas a significant lowering of the concentration of albumin occurs in the serum of women receiving oral contraceptives, a significant increase in the concentration of IgM, ceruloplasmin, and α_1-antitrypsin can be detected. The levels of IgG, IgA, transferrin, and α_2-macroglobulin are similar in the 2 series.

In Table II, the concentrations of the various proteins found at term in the pregnant woman are contrasted with those detected following the use of oral contraceptives. The decrease in albumin concentration and the increase in IgM, ceruloplasmin, and

α_1-antitrypsin noted above in the women taking oral contraceptives also occurs in pregnancy but to a more marked degree. The principle difference in the 2 groups studied is that transferrin is markedly increased in concentration during pregnancy.

Comment

The increasing use of ovarian steroids as an effective and readily accepted contraceptive has quite properly stimulated investigation into their effect on normal physiology. Numerous studies have suggested a similarity to the metabolic alterations detected in normal pregnancy, and in most instances, estrogen rather than any particular progestagen appears to be responsible for the changes produced. Data obtained by Doe, Musa, and Seal[3, 4] indicate a significant elevation in serum ceruloplasmin following estrogen administration which is dose dependent. They also detected an increase in β-glucuronidase, thyroxine-binding globulin, plasminogen, corticosteroid-binding globulin, and 17-hydroxycorticosteroid levels but no changes in sialic acid, transferrin, or hapto-globin levels. Robertson,[6] examining the sera of women taking oral contraceptives with electrophoretic and scanning techniques, noted decreased albumin concentrations and serum cholinesterase levels but increased α_1-globulin concentrations. In the present study, a significant decrease in serum albumin concentration was detected in women using oral contraceptives as well as an increase in the concentration of ceruloplasmin and of α_1-antitrypsin, the principal α_1-globulin in the serum, thus confirming the work of Seal and Robertson. The more marked changes seen in pregnancy at term suggest a dosage-dependency effect, although this phenomenon was not specifically examined in our work. The lack of rise in transferrin concentration following estrogen administration seen in the present study and noted by others[3] is of particular interest in view of the report by Burton[7] that serum total iron-binding capacity is strikingly elevated in the presence of normal transferrin saturation in a group of women using oral contraceptives.

Our knowledge as to the mechanism of production of these alterations is incomplete and controversial. While estrogen has been reported to produce a degree of hemodilution,[8, 9] Robertson's failure to detect hematocrit changes in his study group and the albumin kinetics studies of Hønger[10, 11] suggest that estrogen depresses albumin levels by yet another mechanism. The possibility that a direct effect on hepatic metabolism occurs following estrogen administration stimulated numerous investigations productive of conflicting data. Swyer and Little[12] concluded that there was no evidence of hepatic damage in women taking oral contraceptives for as long as 6 years, while Larsson-Cohn[13] detected abnormal retention of BSP (sulfobromophthalein) in 42 per cent of patients studied. Eisalo, Järvinen, and Luukkainen[14]

also noted abnormal BSP retention in 48 per cent of women receiving a particular oral contraceptive, but among two groups of patients receiving preparations containing a lesser amount of estrogen, no abnormalities were detected. In an investigation of hepatic metabolism of two commonly used anesthetic adjuncts, pethidine and promazine, a diminution in the ability to metabolize these drugs was noted following estrogen and progesterone administration.[15]

The concern over possible alterations in blood coagulation mechanisms with a subsequent predisposition to intravascular clotting following the administration of oral contraceptives, has stimulated numerous laboratory investigations, again with the production of conflicting conclusions. An increase in Factor VII and Factor X has been reported,[16] although Tyler[5] was unable to detect any changes which could be interpreted as demonstrating an increased tendency to spontaneous intravascular clotting. Studies on carbohydrate and lipid metabolism[17, 18] in patients receiving oral contraceptives have demonstrated a significant percentage of patients as having changes resembling those seen in steroid diabetes.

The possibility exists, therefore, that these multiple changes in the concentrations of serum proteins are merely a reflection of altered rates of anabolism and catabolism, and are not indicative of cellular damage. To dismiss the production of these alterations as harmless, however, when continued over the many years encompassing the reproductive period in a woman's life, is open to question. The final judgment awaits the acquisition of additional knowledge about the basic action of ovarian steroids.

The author wishes to acknowledge the excellent technical assistance of Mrs. Julia Deere.

REFERENCES

1. Mendenhall, H. W.: Amer. J. Obstet. Gynec. Accepted for publication.

2. Doe, R. P., Mellinger, G. T., Swain, W. R., and Seal, U. S.: J. Clin. Endocr. 27: 1081, 1967.

3. Musa, B. U., Doe, R. P., and Seal, U. S.: J. Clin. Endocr. **27:** 1463, 1967.
4. Musa, B. U., Seal, U. S., and Doe, R. P.: J. Clin. Endocr. **25:** 1163, 1965.
5. Tyler, E. T.: Brit. Med. J. **2:** 843, 1964.
6. Robertson, G. S.: Lancet **1:** 232, 1967.
7. Burton, J. L.: Lancet **1:** 978, 1967.
8. Witten, C. L., and Bradbury, J. T.: Proc. Soc. Exp. Biol. Med. **78:** 626, 1951.
9. Preedy, J. R. K., and Aitken, E. H.: J. Clin. Invest. **35:** 423, 1956.
10. Hønger, P. E.: Scand. J. Clin. Lab. Invest. **19:** 238, 1967.
11. Hønger, P. E.: Scand. J. Clin. Lab. Invest. **20:** 3, 1967.
12. Swyer, G. I. M., and Little, V.: Brit. Med. J. **1:** 1412, 1965.
13. Larsson-Cohn, U.: Brit. Med. J. **1:** 1414, 1965.
14. Eisalo, A., Järvinen, P. A., and Luukkainen, T.: Brit. Med. J. **1:** 1416, 1965.
15. Crawford, J. S., and Rudofsky, S.: Brit. J. Anaesth. **38:** 446, 1966.
16. Poller, L., and Thomson, J. M.: Brit. Med. J. **2:** 23, 1966.
17. Wynn, V., and Doar, J. W. H.: Lancet **2:** 715, 1966.
18. Wynn, V., and Doar, J. W. H.: Lancet **2:** 720, 1966.

128

Further studies of the effects of an anovulatory drug on lipid metabolism in the rat

L. AFTERGOOD and R. B. ALFIN-SLATER

PREVIOUS REPORTS from our laboratory concerning the effects of contraceptive drugs on lipid metabolism involved the use of large, nonphysiological doses administered to adult female rats fed diets ad lib. Under these conditions, EE given at a level of 1.04 mg (1.0 mg of norethynodrel and 0.04 mg of mestranol) for 4 days resulted in decreased plasma and adrenal cholesterol levels, increased liver cholesterol concentration, and decreased polyunsaturated fatty acids in the cholesteryl esters of plasma and adrenals. Although the treated animals excreted less fecal cholesterol, cholesterol biosynthesis was stimulated in adrenal and ovary but depressed in liver (1, 2).

Abbreviations: EE, Enovid E; HDL, high density lipoproteins.

Recently, several reports relating oral contraceptive therapy to lipid metabolism have appeared in the literature; hypertriglyceridemia, as well as hypercholesterolemia, has been observed in human patients (3–5). It has been suggested (4, 6) that a reduced lipoprotein lipase activity may be a factor contributing to the increased plasma lipid. The activity of this enzyme was found to be influenced in menopausal women by the administration of estrogens (7). Similarly, the lipemia of pregnancy might be due to a diminished uptake of triglyceride fatty acids by the adipose tissue (8). Sachs, Wolfman, and Herzig (9) observed an increase in pre-β-lipoproteins during administration of oral contraceptives and postulated an interference in the formation of β-lipoproteins. Whether these effects would be seen in rats is open to further clarification. In rats, Schweppe and Jungmann (10) observed that whereas low doses of estradiol stimulated in vitro cholesterol esterification in the liver, higher doses antagonized this esterification process.

In the investigation to be reported here, further experiments have been carried out on the effects of EE on lipid metabolism in rats. The dose level of the oral contraceptive was decreased to the amount required for control of fertility. Pair-feeding experiments were also undertaken to eliminate the possibility that the results obtained after hormone administration were due to partial anorexia.

MATERIALS AND METHODS

Female rats of our inbred strain (5–6 months old, avg wt 225 g) were kept on a stock diet of Purina pellets and were administered oral doses of 0.052, 0.52, or 1.04 mg of EE dissolved in sesame seed oil for 4 days before they were killed. In some instances, the rats were put for 4 wk on a high cholesterol diet (1% cholesterol, 0.25% bile salts, and 15% corn oil) prior to being treated with the contraceptive drug. At the end of the experimental period the rats were anesthetized with Nembutal, blood was withdrawn from the heart, and the organs were removed for subsequent analyses.

Cholesterol determinations, thin-layer separations of lipid fractions, and gas–liquid chromatography of fatty

130

acids were performed on various tissues as described previously (1). In this investigation, a Varian Aerograph instrument, Series 200, was used with temperature programming (4°C increase/min from 150°C to 200°C; hydrogen flame detector; the column was packed with 14% Hi-Eff-2BP on Gas-Chrom P, 80–100 mesh). Triglyceride determinations were done using the method of Kaplan and Lee (11); phospholipids were determined by the method of Bartlett (12). Lipoproteins were separated on hydrocellulose gel strips in barbitone acetate buffer with albumin, using a current of 2.5 ma/strip for 45 min. Staining was performed overnight with a saturated solution of Sudan black B in 60% ethanol. Sections of duplicate strips were eluted with acetone and the absorbance of the solution was read at 580 nm.

β-Lipoprotein precipitation from the serum was performed according to the method of Burstein (13).

RESULTS

Experiment I. Pair-feeding Using a Dose Level of 0.52 mg EE

It has been previously observed that rats given doses of 1.04 mg of EE consumed less food than control animals, and lost weight. The possibility that some of the effects of the drug on lipid metabolism could be ascribed to anorexia rather than to the primary hormonal effect required clarification. For this purpose three groups of seven rats each were treated as follows: one group was dosed for 4 days with 0.52 mg EE in sesame oil, two other groups were given sesame oil alone. One of the latter groups of animals was allowed to eat Purina pellets ad lib., while the other group was pair-fed to the drug-treated group. In addition to measuring food consumption and weight gain, feces were collected, dried, and analyzed for cholesterol and total lipid content.

After 4 days of treatment and an overnight fast, rats were killed and serum and liver lipid concentrations were determined. The results are presented in Tables 1–4. As has been reported previously, both serum cholesterol and phospholipid levels were markedly decreased as a result of EE administration; in addition, the choles-

131

terol:phospholipid ratio changed from 0.46 for the control rats to 0.33 for the treated animals. These effects were not secondary to a decreased food consumption. α-Lipoproteins, ordinarily quite abundant in the rat, were very significantly decreased in treated rats; this was verified by the decrease in α/β ratios in these animals (Table 1).

When determinations of cholesterol and phospholipids were made on serum from which β-lipoproteins had been precipitated by heparin and $MnCl_2$, it became obvious that the decrease in cholesterol was primarily in the α-lipoprotein fraction; approximately 90% of this cholesterol disappeared.

There was a significant increase in the weight of the liver of the treated animals (Table 2). Comparisons with pair-fed and ad lib. control groups confirm the fact that these effects are due to the drug and not to changes in food consumption.

Food consumption was markedly reduced, from 8 g per day to 0.5 g per day, as the drug administration progressed; as a result, less feces were excreted by the treated animals (Table 3). Table 4 shows the cholesterol content of feces during EE administration. The cholesterol content of feces was unaffected by diet or treatment with the drug. However, when the average daily excretion of cholesterol was calculated from the total amount of fecal material excreted over the 4-day period, there were noticeable differences between the groups. The treated group excreted less than the ad lib. control ($P < 0.005$) and also less than the pair-fed control ($P < 0.05$).

Experiment II. Comparisons of Results Using Two Dose Levels of EE

In this experiment two levels of EE were used: a dose level equal to the minimum which is effective in preventing conception (14, 15) and a dose which was 10 times higher.

Three groups of adult female rats were treated as follows for 4 days: group 1, sesame oil; group 2, 0.052 mg EE (0.050 mg progestin and 0.002 mg estrogen) in sesame oil; and group 3, 0.52 mg EE (0.50 mg proges-

TABLE 1 EFFECT OF ENOVID E ON CHOLESTEROL AND PHOSPHOLIPIDS IN SERUM AND α-LIPOPROTEINS

| Treatment | Cholesterol | | | Phospholipids | | | C/P | αLP/βLP† |
	Total (C)	αLP (A)	A/C	Total (P)	LP (a)	a/P		
	mg/100 ml		%	*mg/100 ml*		%		
0.52 mg EE	10.8 ± 1.3[ab]*	3.4 ± 0.4[cd]	31.6	32.1 ± 6.2[ef]	29.2 ± 3.4[gh]	91.0	0.33	25/65
Control, pair-fed	41.6 ± 3.6[a]	31.0 ± 2.1[c]	74.5	99.2 ± 10.6[e]	89.5 ± 16.2[α]	90.0	0.41	
Control, ad lib.	46.3 ± 9.9[b]	33.1 ± 2.7[d]	71.5	100.4 ± 15.2[f]	74.9 ± 18.9[h]	75.0	0.46	176/63

Numbers with the *same* letter in superscript are significantly different at $P < 0.001$.

* Mean value ± SD, seven rats per group.

† Ratio of α-lipoprotein to β-lipoprotein as determined by the average absorbance of eluted selections of hydrocellulose gel strips following electrophoresis.

133

TABLE 2 EFFECT OF ENOVID E ON WEIGHT AND CHOLESTEROL CONTENT OF LIVER

Treatment	Liver		Cholesterol in Liver		
	Weight	% Body Wt	Total		% Ester
	g		*mg/g*	*mg/liver*	
0.52 mg EE	5.83 ± 0.46[ad]*	2.78	3.85 ± 0.22[bc]	22.44	43.8
Control, pair-fed	4.91 ± 0.28[a]	2.30	2.42 ± 0.14[b]	11.88	14.0
Control, ad lib.	4.85 ± 0.27[d]	2.26	2.38 ± 0.08[c]	11.54	13.5

Numbers with the *same* letter in superscript are significantly different; superscripts a–c indicate significant difference at $P < 0.001$, and d, at $P < 0.005$.
* Mean value ± SD, seven rats per group.

TABLE 3 EFFECT OF ENOVID E ON FOOD CONSUMPTION AND EXCRETION OF FECES

Treatment	Day 1		Day 2		Day 3		Day 4*	
	Food Ingested	Feces Excreted	Food Ingested	Feces Excreted	Food Ingested	Feces Excreted	Food Ingested	Feces Excreted
	g	*g†*	*g*	*g†*	*g*	*g†*	*g*	*g†*
0.52 mg EE	8 ± 1‡	1.33 ± 0.80	6 ± 1	1.02 ± 0.41[a]§	4 ± 1	0.79 ± 0.26[bc]	0.5 ± 0.8	0.90 ± 0.31[d]
Control, pair-fed	9 ± 2	1.73 ± 0.38	6 ± 1	1.66 ± 0.43	4 ± 1	1.45 ± 0.45[b]	1.0 ± 1.0	0.74 ± 0.26
Control, ad lib.	11 ± 2	1.25 ± 0.39	10 ± 2	2.02 ± 0.72[a]	12 ± 2	2.00 ± 0.58[c]	2.0 ± 0.7	1.79 ± 0.47[d]

* Food was removed from cages 16 hr before the rats were killed.
† Dry weight.
‡ Mean value ± SD, seven rats per group.
§ Superscripts a and b indicate significant difference at $P < 0.01$, and c and d, at $P < 0.005$. Numbers with *same* letter in superscript are significantly different.

TABLE 4   Effect of Enovid E on Excretion of Cholesterol in the Feces

Treatment	Cholesterol Excretion				Average Daily Excretion, Day 1–4	Fecal Cholesterol, Day 1–4
	Day 1	Day 2	Day 3	Day 4		
	mg/rat/day				*mg/rat*	*mg/g*
0.52 mg EE	4.1 ± 2.4*	4.2 ± 1.1	3.0 ± 1.1	2.7 ± 2.0	3.5 ± 0.4[ab]†	3.3
Control, pair-fed	6.3 ± 2.0	4.9 ± 1.3	4.5 ± 2.3	2.8 ± 0.3	4.6 ± 0.7[a]	3.4
Control, ad lib.	4.0 ± 1.3	6.1 ± 2.2	5.8 ± 1.6	3.5 ± 1.6	5.1 ± 0.5[b]	3.0

* Mean value ± sd, seven rats per group.
† Numbers with superscripts a and b are significantly different at $P < 0.05$ and $P < 0.005$, respectively.

tin and 0.02 mg estrogen in sesame oil). The rats were killed following an overnight fast. It can be seen (Table 5) that even at the low physiological dose (0.052 mg) of EE, there were marked changes in lipid levels; in serum, cholesterol decreased from 47.8 to 15.5 mg per 100 ml and phospholipid decreased from 118.5 to 62.8 mg per 100 ml. The C/P and the α/β lipoprotein ratios also decreased. Higher doses of the drug enhanced most of these changes.

In liver (Table 6), the triglyceride levels were decreased and the cholesterol content was increased following hormonal treatment. No changes were observed in the phospholipids even when the larger dose level, 0.52 mg of EE, was administered.

Table 7 shows the fatty acid composition of the liver cholesteryl esters and the concentration of individual cholesteryl esters. The decrease of arachidonate observed in those animals receiving the larger dose of EE was accompanied by an increase of oleate. However, taking into account the concentration of liver cholesteryl esters (Table 6), the actual amount of cholesteryl arachidonate did not change while other esters increased appreciably.

Experiment III. Effects of Various Levels of EE on Cholesterol-fed Rats

In this experiment adult female rats were fed a high cholesterol diet for 4 wk. The animals were then divided into three groups, and they were given diets supplemented with sesame oil, 0.52 mg EE in sesame oil, or 1.04 mg EE in sesame oil, for 4 days. The results of the lipid analyses performed on these animals are shown in Tables 8–10.

There was a marked decrease in serum total cholesterol levels as well as in serum triglyceride levels (Table 8). Both doses of the drug exerted rather similar effects, although a significant decrease in triglyceride values was not achieved until the larger dose was administered. The amount of cholesteryl esters in the serum decreased, with arachidonate being lowered more than the other cholesteryl esters. The ovarian cholesterol content did not change when expressed as per gram of tissue (Table 9). However, the size of the ovary decreased as a result of EE administration and therefore total cholesterol

TABLE 5 EFFECT OF DOSE OF ENOVID E ON SERUM CHOLESTEROL AND PHOSPHOLIPIDS

Treatment	Cholesterol			Phospholipids (P)	C/P	αLP/βLP*
	Total (C)	Free	% Ester			
	mg/100 ml			*mg/100 ml*		
Control	47.8 ± 5.4†ᵃ	15.9 ± 2.9ᵇ	66.7	118.5 ± 13.2ᶜ	0.40	165/64ᵈᵉ
0.052 mg EE	15.5 ± 3.6ᵃ	4.8 ± 0.4ᵇ	69.0	62.8 ± 11.4ᶜ	0.25	19/56ᵈ
0.52 mg EE	4.2 ± 1.9ᵃ	2.0 ± 0.9ᵇ	52.5	23.6 ± 4.7ᶜ	0.18	26/69ᵉ

Numbers with the *same* letter in superscript are significantly different at the following levels: a, b, and c, $P < 0.001$; d, $P < 0.025$; and e, $P < 0.01$.

* See footnote (†) to Table 1.

† Mean value ± SD, six rats per group.

TABLE 6 EFFECT OF DOSE OF ENOVID E ON LIVER LIPIDS

Treatment	Liver		Cholesterol				Phospholipids	Triglycerides
	Weight	% Body Wt	Total		Ester	% Ester		
	g		*mg/g*	*mg/organ*	*mg/g*		*mg/g*	*mg/g*
Control	5.80 ± 0.32*	2.46	2.48 ± 0.12ᵃᶜ†	14.38	0.31 ± 0.15ᵈ	12.5	25.8 ± 3.8	17.2 ± 6.8ᶠᵍ
0.052 mg EE	6.06 ± 0.66	2.55	2.84 ± 0.33ᵃᵇ	17.21	0.59 ± 0.35ᵉ	20.8	23.8 ± 8.2	8.9 ± 2.9ᶠ
0.52 mg EE	6.01 ± 0.73	2.73	3.31 ± 0.24ᵇᶜ	19.88	1.00 ± 0.23ᵈᵉ	30.0	24.9 ± 11.8	7.5 ± 0.7ᵍ

* Mean value ± SD, six rats per group.

† Numbers with the *same* letter in superscript are significantly different at the following levels: a, e, and f, $P < 0.05$; b and g, $P < 0.025$; c, $P < 0.001$; and d, $P < 0.005$.

TABLE 7 EFFECT OF DOSE OF ENOVID E ON FATTY ACID
COMPOSITION AND CONCENTRATION OF CHOLESTERYL ESTERS
IN THE LIVER

	Control	Treatment	
		0.052 mg EE	0.52 mg EE
16:0*	29.1 ± 4.3†	27.5 ± 3.7	24.8 ± 2.5
	(9)‡	(16)	(25)
16:1	5.8 ± 1.5	6.5 ± 1.4	7.4 ± 2.9
	(2)	(4)	(7)
18:0	9.5 ± 0.7	9.8 ± 1.6	7.3 ± 1.6
	(3)	(6)	(7)
18:1	16.4 ± 2.1[ab]§	23.4 ± 2.6[a]	29.4 ± 3.5[b]
	(5)	(14)	(29)
18:2	10.9 ± 1.7	11.4 ± 1.7	14.2 ± 1.4
	(3)	(7)	(14)
20:4	15.1 ± 1.7[cd]	8.3 ± 0.9[c]	6.3 ± 1.8[d]
	(5)	(5)	(6)

* No. of carbon atoms : no. of double bonds.

† % of total cholesteryl ester fatty acids, mean ± SD, six rats per group.

‡ Values in parentheses are concentrations (mg/g of liver) of individual cholesteryl esters.

§ Numbers with the *same* letter in superscript are significantly different at $P < 0.001$.

was depressed when expressed as the cholesterol content of the whole organ. Adrenal cholesterol (per gram of tissue or per gland) was decreased by EE administration.

The effect of the drug on liver lipids (Table 10) of cholesterol-fed rats differed from what was observed in rats fed stock diets. Since a large amount of cholesterol accumulated in the liver as a result of cholesterol feeding, the increase in hepatic cholesterol resulting from drug administration for 4 days was masked and was not significant. However, the triglyceride concentration was markedly decreased (from 25.14 to 9.30 mg/g).

TABLE 8 Effect of Dose of Enovid E on Serum Lipids in Cholesterol-fed Rats

Treatment	Cholesterol		Cholesteryl			Triglycerides
	Total	Esterified	Oleate	Linoleate	Arachi-donate	
	$mg/100\,ml$			$mg/100\,ml$		$mg/100\,ml$
Control	125.1 ± 25.0*[ab]	93.1 ± 7.1[cd]	19	22	29	40.1 ± 18.3[e]
0.52 mg EE	57.4 ± 16.8[a]	33.7 ± 7.7[c]	9	9	7	20.9 ± 10.9
1.04 mg EE	59.4 ± 20.3[b]	39.1 ± 6.1[d]	10	10	5	14.7 ± 11.6[e]

Numbers with the *same* letter in superscript are significantly different; superscripts a–d indicate significant difference at $P < 0.001$, and e, at $P < 0.025$.

* Mean value ± sᴅ, six rats per group.

139

DISCUSSION

The results of the first experiment have confirmed our previous findings that lipid metabolism of female rats is significantly affected by the administration of an oral contraceptive drug. In these experiments, a much lower dose than the one used previously also resulted in reduced serum cholesterol and phospholipid levels and increased cholesteryl esters in the liver. It has been shown that these effects were not secondary to a decreased food consumption. Cholesterol excretion was decreased in

TABLE 9 EFFECT OF DOSE OF ENOVID E ON ADRENAL AND CVARY CHOLESTEROL IN CHOLESTEROL-FED RATS*

Treatment	Cholesterol in Adrenals		Cholesterol in Ovaries	
	mg/g	$mg/organ$	mg/g	$mg/organ$
Control	62.4	2.86	12.8	0.42
0.52 mg EE	37.2	1.94	12.8	0.34
1.04 mg EE	33.2	1.63	12.4	0.33

* Analyses were carried out on pooled organs.

animals given the oral contraceptive drug. Although fecal cholesterol determinations are of limited value in appraising cholesterol balance, the fact that the treated animals fed a cholesterol-free diet excreted less cholesterol or its metabolities, or both, than the untreated animals should be accepted at least as an indication of some change in cholesterol metabolism. We have previously observed more highly significant differences in fecal sterol excretion when higher doses of the drug were administered (2).

Since most of the phospholipids are present in the α-lipoproteins, the effect observed in total serum phospholipids was clearly reflected by decreases in phospholipids of α-lipoprotein. However, the phospholipids were not decreased at the same rate as cholesterol since the resulting cholesterol:phospholipid ratio was depressed. Hill and Dvornik (16) have also shown a fall in the cholesterol:phospholipid ratio in lipoproteins as a result of estradiol-17-β administration to male rats.

In the second experiment reported here, physiological doses of the drug (with antifertility activity) also resulted in deviations from "normal" cholesterol metabolism.

140

TABLE 10 Effect of Dose of Enovid E on Liver Lipids in Cholesterol-fed Rats

Treatment	Liver		Total Lipids	Cholesterol			Triglycerides
	Weight	% Body Wt		Total		Free	
	g		*mg/g*	*mg/g*	*mg/organ*	*mg/g*	*mg/g*
Control	8.00 ± 1.03*	3.3	106.5 ± 2.38	19.50 ± 6.03	15.60	3.30 ± 0.79	25.14 ± 5.13[a,b]†
0.052 mg EE	7.79 ± 1.02	3.2	100.9 ± 13.8	20.53 ± 3.66	15.99	3.94 ± 0.65	10.85 ± 2.97[a]
1.04 mg EE	7.74 ± 0.78	3.3	85.9 ± 13.4	22.32 ± 2.43	17.27	3.87 ± 0.45	9.30 ± 4.57[b]

* Mean value ± SD, six rats per group.
† Numbers with the *same* letter in superscript are significantly different at $P < 0.001$.

The dose levels used here were 1/10 of the amount which had produced responses in our previous experiments.

The effect of contraceptive drugs on serum lipoprotein levels has also been shown in other investigations. According to Furman (17), estrogen administration to humans diminishes the cholesterol content of α-lipoproteins relative to phospholipid and protein content, and increases the concentration of α-lipoproteins in the serum. Horne, Howie, Weir, and Goudie (18) found elevated serum levels of α-macroglobulin in women taking oral contraceptives.

Mendenhall (19) has reported decreases in albumin and increases in immunoglobulin, ceruloplasmin, and α-antitrypsin in women taking oral contraceptives. Similar, more marked changes have been observed in pregnant women at term.

We have previously reported an enhancement of lecithin–cholesterol acyltransferase activity in plasma of rats treated with the contraceptive drug (1). This enzyme has been shown to be associated with HDL (20). As suggested by Rowen and Martin (21), the disruption of HDL structure exposes lipids to the transferase enzyme with resulting enhancement of its activity.

In the first two experiments reported here cholesteryl esters accumulated in the liver (Tables 2 and 6). The fatty acids esterified with cholesterol were primarily palmitic, oleic, and linoleic; the total amount of cholesteryl arachidonate did not change appreciably, although the proportion of cholesteryl arachidonate decreased considerably as the other esters increased. It has been suggested by Gidez, Roheim, and Eder (22) that there is a preferential incorporation of cholesteryl esters of polyenoic acids into the HDL. The reduction of serum HDL rich in highly unsaturated esters would result in a reduced amount of unsaturated cholesteryl esters. We have previously reported that, in plasma, there was a decrease in cholesteryl arachidonate and linoleate with corresponding increases of palmitate, palmitoleate, stearate, and oleate when 1.04 mg EE was administered (1).

The fact that cholesteryl arachidonate does not accumulate in the liver may mean that its incorporation into HDL and the subsequent turnover of HDL must be

142

quite rapid. On the other hand, there might be an interference with arachidonate biosynthesis from linoleate; the linoleate content in the liver increases as the dose level of the drug increases. The fact that there are very definite changes in fatty acid pattern of cholesteryl esters both in the serum and in the liver denies the theory of simple redistribution of cholesterol within the body. Obviously, it would seem that cholesteryl arachidonate is being preferentially metabolized.

It has been shown previously that cholesteryl esters act as a reservoir of steroid precursors. Most of the cholesterol in rat adrenal glands is esterified; the fatty acids characteristically contain high percentages of the tetraenoic acids (20:4 and 22:4) (23). Sayers, Sayers, White, and Long (24) showed that administration of ACTH to rats caused a depletion of cholesterol in the adrenal. Recently, Gidez and Feller (25) have shown that a unilateral adrenalectomy causes a selective decrease of cholesteryl arachidonate in the remaining organ. They suggest that selectivity in the depletion of cholesteryl esters is due to differences in their rates of hydrolysis. Apparently, hydrolysis of esters must precede the conversion. In dog adrenals, hydrolysis of esters could be demonstrated as well as synthesis of labeled steroids from cholesterol esters (26).

It has been shown (27) that adrenals are among the most active tissues capable of removing cholesteryl esters from plasma. This process may also be instrumental in supplying cholesterol for further metabolism in these glands (in addition to stimulated biosynthesis) while at the same time being responsible for reduction of cholesterol in plasma.

In an organ overloaded with exogenous cholesterol (experiment III), the effects of the drug were somewhat masked. However, even under these conditions hypolipemic action was observed after drug administration. Here again serum cholesteryl arachidonate was decreased to the greatest extent.

It is possible that the short-term effects of anovulatory drugs may be modified by long-term administration. Studies in which physiological doses of these compounds or their components are given to adult animals over their life span are in order at this time.

143

Partial support from the Research Committee of the UCLA School of Public Health is hereby gratefully acknowledged.

REFERENCES

1. Aftergood, L., H. J. Hernandez, and R. B. Alfin-Slater. 1968. Effect of large doses of the oral contraceptive Enovid on cholesterol metabolism in the rat. *J. Lipid Res.* **9:** 447–452.
2. Alfin-Slater, R. B., and L. Aftergood. 1968. The effect of a steroid anti-ovulatory agent on cholesterol metabolism in rats. *Proc. West. Hemisphere Nutr. Congr. II.* 253.
3. Zorilla, E., M. Hulse, A. Hernandez, and H. Gershberg. 1968. Severe endogenous hypertriglyceridemia during treatment with estrogen and oral contraceptives. *J. Clin. Endocrinol. Metab.* **28:** 1793–1797.
4. Hazzard, W. R., M. J. Spiger, J. D. Bagdade, and E. L. Bierman. 1969. Studies on the mechanism of increased plasma triglyceride levels induced by oral contraceptives. *N. Engl. J. Med.* **280:** 471–476.
5. Wynn, V., J. W. H. Doar, G. L. Mills, and T. Stokes. 1969. Fasting serum triglycerides, cholesterol and lipoprotein levels during oral contraceptive therapy. *Lancet.* **2:** 756–760.
6. Ham, J. M., and R. Rose. 1969. Platelet adhesiveness and lipoprotein lipase activity in controls and in subjects taking oral contraceptives. *Amer. J. Obstet. Gynecol.* **105:** 628–631.
7. Fabian, E., A. Štork, J. Kobilková, and J. Šponarová. 1967. The activity of the lipoprotein lipase and estrogens. *Enzymol. Biol. Clin.* **8:** 451–455.
8. Otway, S., and D. S. Robinson. 1968. The significance of changes in tissue clearing factor lipase activity in relation to the lipaemia of pregnancy. *Biochem. J.* **106:** 677–682.
9. Sachs, B. A., L. Wolfman, and N. Herzig. 1969. Plasma lipid and lipoprotein alterations during oral contraceptive administration. *Obstet. Gynecol.* **34:** 530–534.
10. Schweppe, J. S., and R. A. Jungmann. 1969. The effect of hormones on hepatic cholesterol ester synthesis in vitro. *Proc. Soc. Exp. Biol. Med.* **131:** 868–870.
11. Kaplan, A., and V. F. Lee. 1965. A micromethod for determination of serum triglycerides. *Proc. Soc. Exp. Biol. Med.* **118:** 296–297.
12. Bartlett, G. R. 1959. Phosphorus assay in column chromatography. *J. Biol. Chem.* **234:** 466–468.
13. Burstein, M. 1960. Dosage du cholestérol dans les α et les β lipoprotéines du serum par une methode basée sur la precipitation sélective des β lipoprotéines. *Pathol. Biol.* **8:** 1247–1249.
14. Yang, M. G., V. L. Sanger, and O. Mickelsen. 1969. Feeding norethynodrel and mestranol to immature and adult female rats. *Proc. Soc. Exp. Biol. Med.* **130:** 1146–1149.

15. Banik, U. K., C. Revesz, and F. Herr. 1969. Orally active estrogens and progestins in prevention of pregnancy in rats. *J. Reprod. Fert.* **18:** 509–513.
16. Hill, P., and D. Dvornik. 1969. Agents affecting lipid metabolism. XXXVII. Separation of rat serum lipoproteins with dextran sulfate. *Can. J. Biochem.* **47:** 1043–1048.
17. Furman, R. H. 1969. Gonadal steroid effects on serum lipids. *In* Metabolic Effects of Gonadal Hormones and Contraceptive Steroids. H. A. Salhanick, editor. Plenum Press, N.Y. 247–264.
18. Horne, C. H. W., P. W. Howie, R. J. Weir, and R. B. Goudie. 1970. Effect of combined estrogen-progestogen oral contraceptives on serum-levels of α_2 macroglobulin, transferrin, albumin, and IgG. *Lancet.* **1:** 49–50.
19. Mendenhall, H. W. 1970. Effect of oral contraceptives on serum protein concentrations. *Amer. J. Obstet. Gynecol.* **106:** 750–753.
20. Lossow, W. J., S. N. Shah, and I. L. Chaikoff. 1966. Isolation of cholesterol-esterifying activity in rat serum by ultracentrifugal flotation. *Biochim. Biophys. Acta.* **116:** 172–174.
21. Rowen, R., and J. Martin. 1963. Enhancement of cholesterol esterification in serum by an extract of group A Streptococcus. *Biochim. Biophys. Acta.* **70:** 396–405.
22. Gidez, L. I., P. S. Roheim, and H. A. Eder. 1965. Effect of diet on the cholesterol ester composition of liver and of plasma lipoproteins in the rat. *J. Lipid Res.* **6:** 377–382.
23. Gidez, L. I. 1964. Occurrence of a docosatrienoic acid in the cholesterol esters of adrenals of rats on EFA deficient diet. *Biochem. Biophys. Res. Commun.* **14:** 413–418.
24. Sayers, G., M. A. Sayers, A. White, and C. N. H. Long. 1943. Effect of pituitary adrenotropic hormone on cholesterol content of rat adrenal glands. *Proc. Soc. Exp. Biol. Med.* **52:** 200–202.
25. Gidez, L. I., and E. Feller. 1969. Effect of the stress of unilateral adrenalectomy on the depletion of individual cholesteryl esters in the rat adrenal. *J. Lipid Res.* **10:** 656–659.
26. Dailey, R. E., L. Swell, and C. R. Treadwell. 1963. Hydrolysis and utilization of cholesterol esters for steroid synthesis by canine adrenal homogenates. *Arch. Biochem. Biophys.* **100:** 360–363.
27. Brot, N., W. J. Lossow, and I. L. Chaikoff. 1964. In vitro uptake and hydrolysis, by rat tissues, of cholesterol esters of a very low density, chyle lipoprotein fraction. *J. Lipid Res.* **5:** 63–67.

Effect of ovarian steroids on hepatic metabolism

II. Estrogens

M. S. FAHIM, Ph.D.

D. G. HALL, M.D.

T. JONES, B.S.

As MORE AND MORE of the world's female population consumes oral contraceptive drugs, increasing concern is developing as to the possibility of hazardous side effects. Since the liver is well known to be the primary organ by which the biotransformation and inactivation of certain hormones take place, it is possible that drug-induced metabolic interactions might well influence directly or indirectly the homeostasis of hepatic function. Particularly relevant in this connection is the fact that the metabolic conversion of steroids by means of reduction, hydroxylation, oxidation, and conjugation has a manyfold biologic effect on the liver.

It has been demonstrated that progesterone affects sexually mature female rats in a manner similar to phenobarbital, causing increased liver weight, hepatic demethylation, hepatic microsomal protein, and excretion of ascorbic acid in the urine. Although progesterone appears to function as an hepatic enzyme inducer in adult female rats, a re-

verse effect is noted in males.[1] In rats, urinary excretion of ascorbic acid is used as an index of hepatic enzyme activity, since compounds that increase the activity of microsomal enzymes stimulate the metabolism of glucose and galactose via the glucuronic acid pathway through D-glucuronic acid and L-gluconic acid to ascorbic acid.

In human beings, a similar acceleration in the synthesis of D-glucaric acid has been demonstrated in postmenopausal women. The administration of 50 mg. of progesterone daily for 3 days resulted in a significant elevation of urinary D-glucaric acid.[2]

The present study was designed to evaluate the effect of natural and synthetic estrogens on the hepatic nicotinamide adenine dinucleotide phosphate (NADPH) oxygen-dependent "drug-metabolizing" reduced enzymes in sexually mature female and male rats.

Material and methods

Two hundred sexually mature female and male rats of the Holtzman strain, maintained in a controlled temperature of $25.5 \pm 1.0^\circ$ C., were divided into 9 groups. Group 1 consisted of 20 males and 20 females, and Groups 2 through 9 consisted of 10 males and 10 females: Group 1, control; Group 2, 1γ 17β-estradiol daily; Group 3, 100Υ 17β-

Supported by the National Institutes of Health General Medical Science Grant No. PH 43-68-952 and Medical School Research Fund in Reproductive Biology, No. 258-295.

146

estradiol daily; Group 4, 1γ diethylstilbestrol daily; Group 5, 100γ diethylstilbestrol daily; Group 6, 100 γ chlorotrianisene daily; Group 7, 1 mg. chlorotrianisene daily; Group 8, 100γ clomiphene citrate daily; Group 9, 1 mg. clomiphene citrate daily.

The estrogens were administered subcutaneously daily for 10 days. On the eleventh day, the animals were decapitated, and the livers were immediately removed, rinsed, blotted, and homogenized in 3 volumes of 1.15 per cent KCl in a potter-Elvehjem glass homogenizer. The liver homogenates were centrifuged at 9,000 g in a refrigerated Sorvall centrifuge for 20 minutes, and the supernatant was decanted and stored at $-20°$ C. until assayed for enzymatic demethylation of P-chloro-N-methylaniline according to the Kupfer and Bruggeman[3] technique.

All data were evaluated statistically by analysis of variance, and the least significant difference was determined.[4]

Results

Natural estrogen (17β-estradiol). Treatment of female and male rats with 17β-estradiol resulted in a significant decrease (P <0.01) in the rate of hepatic demethylation (Table I). In females treated with 1γ and 100γ doses, the reduction was 18.56 and 34.75 per cent, respectively, compared to the control animals (Fig. 1). Values for similarly treated males decreased 36.61 and 42.21 per cent (Fig. 2).

Nonsteroid estrogens

Diethylstilbestrol. Both female and male animals demonstrated a significant reduction (P <0.01) of hepatic demethylation activity (Table I). Females receiving 1γ and 100γ exhibited a reduction of hepatic enzymatic activity of 21.25 and 23.86 per cent, as compared to control groups (Fig. 1). In males, a reduction of 38.06 and 41.11 per cent was noted (Fig. 2).

Chlorotrianisene. It is interesting to note that administration of chlorotrianisene to female rats resulted in a significant increase of hepatic demethylation (P <0.01), while

Table I. Effect of estrogens on hepatic demethylation in female and male rats

Treatment	Female (mm. PCA/ gram)*	Male (mm. PCA/ gram)*
Control	1.341 ± 0.071	2.685 ± 0.084
17β-estradiol, 1 γ	1.092 ± 0.046	1.702 ± 0.053
17β-estradiol, 100 γ	0.875 ± 0.065	1.553 ± 0.061
Stilbestrol, 1 γ	1.056 ± 0.084	1.663 ± 0.037
Stilbestrol, 100 γ	1.021 ± 0.074	1.581 ± 0.063
Chlorotrianisene, 100 γ	1.738 ± 0.051	1.992 ± 0.078
Chlorotrianisene, 1 mg.	1.665 ± 0.079	1.772 ± 0.049
Clomiphene citrate, 100 γ	1.864 ± 0.063	2.584 ± 0.064
Clomiphene citrate, 1 mg.	1.926 ± 0.048	2.791 ± 0.049

± = standard error.
*PCA = P-chloro-n-methylaniline.

the reverse occurred in males (Table I). Female rats treated with 100γ and 1 mg. chlorotrianisene increased their hepatic microsomal activity 29.69 and 24.16 per cent (Fig. 1), as compared to controls, while that of similarly treated males decreased 25.81 and 34.00 per cent (Fig. 2).

Clomiphene citrate. Female rats treated with clomiphene citrate showed a significant increase in hepatic activity (P <0.01). The increase was 39.00 per cent for groups receiving 100γ and 43.62 for those receiving 1 mg. (Fig. 1). Males receiving clomiphene citrate exhibited no significant variation in hepatic demethylation.

Comment

It has been frequently demonstrated that a large variety of substances are metabolized by mixed-function oxidases localized in the endoplasmic reticulum of the liver. Brodie and associates,[5] in 1958, demonstrated that the hepatic microsomal NADPH-linked enzyme system is a common pathway for the hydroxylation of a variety of drugs and other aromatic compounds.

In this investigation, we assayed the rate of demethylation of the aromatic amine (P-chloroaniline) by liver microsomal systems as a measure of the activity of NADPH-oxygen–dependent "drug-metabolizing" enzymes.[4]

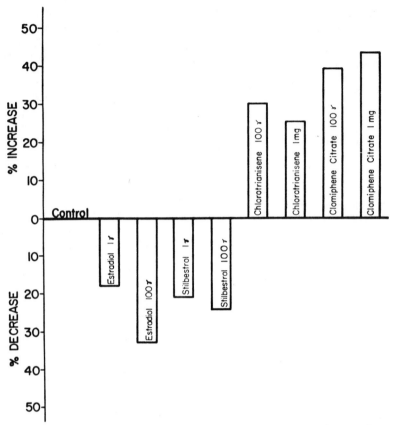

Fig. 1. Effect of estrogens on hepatic demethylation in female rats as compared to control.

Recently Palmer and colleagues[6] indicated that the administration of natural estrogens (estradiol, estrone, and estriol) and synthetic estrogens (estradiol-3-acetate, estradiol-17-acetate, and estradiol-3-methyl ether) impairs the biliary excretion of sulfobromophthalein in rats.[6]

The results of this study indicate that 17β-estradiol produces a state of hepatic inhibition when administered to sexually mature male and female rats.

Inscoe and Axelrod[7] noted that estradiol reduced the glucuronyl transferase activity in liver microsomes of male rats.

The results of this investigation indicate that a nonsteroid estrogen (diethylstilbestrol) reduces hepatic demethylation activity in both female and male rats.

Chlorotrianisene and clomiphene citrate, derivatives of diethylstilbestrol, stimulate hepatic demethylation in female rats. In males, however, chlorotrianisene acts as an enzyme inhibitor while clomiphene citrate exerts a neutral effect. These observations suggest that the effect of estrogens on hepatic function relates both to the structural characteristics of the estrogens and the sex of the recipient.

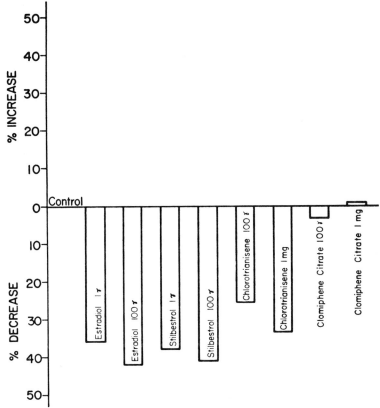

Fig. 2. Effect of estrogen treatment on hepatic demethylation in male rats as compared to controls.

Zumoff and co-workers[8] investigated the peripheral metabolism of tracer quantities of radioactive estradiol in normal young and elderly adult men and women. The fraction of hormone metabolite recovered in the urine and the pattern of conjugation of these metabolites were found to be influenced by age and sex whereas the fraction recovered as "glucosiduronates" and the distribution of metabolites within the "glucosiduronate fraction" were independent of age and sex.[9]

Oral contraceptives are combinations of synthetic progestins and estrogens in ratios of 10:1 or greater. Most available reports indicate that impairment of the bile secretory function of liver cell as measured by sulfobromophthalein retention occurs in 5 to 40 per cent of patients taking these preparations.[10-14]

In general, sulfobromophthalein retention appears closely related to progestogen dosage, but in individual patients increased doses do not necessarily increase sulfobromophthalein retention.

Retention of sulfobromophthalein, as all function test abnormalities to be described, is often transient and may eventually disappear despite continued drug adiministration.[15-16]

Recently, we have demonstrated that natural progesterone acts as an enzyme inducer in female rats and postmenopausal women.[1-2]

To elucidate the relationship between estrogens and progesterone and intrahepatic cholestasis, studies of hepatic function have been made in a susceptible subject treated with a variety of natural and synthetic estrogenic and progestational compounds.[17] This patient had previously developed intrahepatic cholestatic jaundice during each of three pregnancies and also following the ingestion on norethynodrel-mestranol.* Oral treatment with the natural agent, progesterone, 10 mg. per day for one week, and with the synthetic progestogens, medroxy-progesterone acetate, 10 mg. per day for one week, and 17-α-ethynyloestrenol, 10 mg. per day for 5 days, was not followed by any alteration in hepatic function as assessed by serum bilirubin concentration, serum activities of glutamic-pyruvic transaminase, glutamic-oxalacetic transaminase, lactic dehydrogenase, sulfobromophthalein retention, or cephalic flocculation. Oral treatment with natural estrogens, equilin and estrone, 2.5 mg. per day for 21 days, and estradiol, 1.5 mg. per day for 14 days, produced hepatic dysfunction with pruritus, nausea, increase in serum activities of glutamic-pyruvic transaminase, glutamic-oxalacetic transaminase, lactic dehydrogenase, and sulfobromophthalein retention. Stilbestrol, 0.02 mg per day, produced nausea and pruritis after 9 days, with biochemical evidence of hepatic dysfunction.[17]

*Enovid, G. A. Searle & Co., Chicago, Illinois.

These findings support the view that intrahepatic cholestasis of pregnancy and jaundice secondary to antifertility drugs are caused by estrogenic rather than progestational activity.

There are 22 brands of the pill marketed in the United States, each differing in the type and quantitation of component hormones. These brands contain 2 types of estrogen, mestranol, and ethinyl estradiol, and 7 progestational agents, norethynodrel, norethindrone, norethindrone acetate, medroxyprogesterone, chlormadinone acetate, ethynodial diacetate, and norgestrel.

Contraceptive drugs are far from being identical or interchangeable. They differ biologically, physiologically and pharmacologically. Modern chemical ingenuity has synthesized a vast array of steroid molecules and produced a comparatively thorough understanding of their chemical characteristics.

Little, however, is known of their metabolic interactions or effect on bodily homeostasis. It has long been recognized that certain steroids, particularly those with an alkylated group at C17 are hepatotoxic.[18-22] Results of the present investigation also indicate that the effect of steroids on hepatic activity is structurally related.

Clarification of the acute and long-range hepatic response to the components of currently available oral antifertility drugs is not only pertinent but might well facilitate modifications leading to improved drug contraception.

We acknowledge the William S. Merrill Company for supplying clomiphene citrate and TACE for this investigation.

REFERENCES

1. Fahim, M. S., and Hall, D. G.: AMER. J. OBSTET. GYNEC. 106: 183, 1970.
2. Fahim, M. S., Hall. D. G., and Fahim. Z.: AMER. J. OBSTET. GYNEC. 105: 124, 1969.
3. Kupfer, D., and Bruggeman, L. L.: Anal. Biochem. 17: 502, 1966.
4. Snedecor, G. W.: Statistical Methods, ed. 5, Ames, Iowa 1956, Low University Press.
5. Brodie, B. B., Gillette, J. R., and LaDu, B. N.: Ann. Rev. Biochem. 27: 27, 1958.
6. Palmer, R. H., Gallagher, T. J., Jr., Mueller, M. N., and Kapps, A.: In Salhanic, H. A., Kipnis, D. M., and Wiele, R. L., editors: Metabolic Effects of Gonadal Hormones and Contraceptive Steroids, New York, 1969, Plenum Press Inc., p. 19.
7. Inscoe, J. K., and Axelrod, J.: J. Pharmacol. Exp. Ther. 129: 128, 1960.
8. Zumoff, B., Fishman, J., Gallagher, T., and Hellman, L.: J. Clin. Endocr. 28: 937, 1968.
9. Ramanoff, L. P., Rodriguez, R. M., Seelye, J. M., Parent, C., and Pincus, C.: J. Clin. Endocr. 18: 1255, 1958.
10. Tuler, E. T.: Brit. Med. J. 2: 283, 1964.
11. Linthorst, G.: Brit. Med. J. 2: 920, 1964.

12. Borglin, N. E.: Brit. Med. J. 1: 1280, 1965.
13. Larrson-Cohn, U.: Brit. Med. J. 1: 1414, 1965.
14. Eisentadt, H. B.: J. A. M. A. 194: 933, 1965.
15. Goldzieher, J. W.: Med. Clin. N. Amer. 48: 529, 1964.
16. Ricewory, E.: Brit. Med. J. 2: 1011, 1964.
17. Boake, W. C.: Acta. Endocr. 119: 169, 1967 (Suppl.).

18. Drill, V. A.: Fed. Proc. 18: 1040, 1959.
19. Mueller, M. M., and Kappas, A.: J. Clin. Invest. 43: 1905, 1964.
20. Ockner, R. K., and Davidson, C. S.: New Eng. J. Med. 276: 331, 1967.
21. Schaffner, F.: J. A. M. A. 198: 1019, 1966.
22. Sherlock, S.: Diseases of the Liver, Philadelphia, 1963, F. A. Davis Company, p. 307.

Social and Psychological Effects Attributed
to Oral Contraceptives

SIDE EFFECTS OF ORAL CONTRACEPTIVE MEDICATION:
A PSYCHOSOMATIC PROBLEM

J. N. FORTIN, M.D. , E. D. WITTKOWER, M.D. , J. PAIEMENT, M.D. and
L. TETREAULT, M.D.

The widespread use of oral contraceptive medication raises many problems, and the abundant literature on the subject, describing the multi-varied effects of its use, requires dispassionate assessment. This report explores the relevance of emotional factors to the appearance of side effects and the manner in which the emotional factors operate. These potent therapeutic agents have contributed to 'diseases of medical progress', as is indicated by many clinical and experimental reports.

Because the primary objective of this medication is contraception all phenomena other than contraception, be they biological or psychological, set in motion by and occurring concomitantly with the administration of the drug, can be regarded as side effects. These phenomena are studied in the light of new perspectives in psychosomatic medicine (9).

Previous Studies

The available literature on the subject, illustrating the interests of investigators from many countries, ranges from a discussion of the serious side effects of the medication as such to the emotional forces affecting the attitudes of men and women toward it. A complete survey has become a monumental task, and only the literature which focuses on the topic under present study will be reviewed.

Bakker and Dightman (1), with data involving one hundred couples on norethylno-drel, reported that weight gain and depression were considered a 'scapegoat effect'. Fluid retention was a significant problem in 30 per cent of their subjects and was pharmacologically-induced as an 'all or none' effect. There was no indication whatsoever that loss of libido was a *bona fide* side effect.

Glick (2) in his extensive survey emphasized that there is not sufficient evidence upon which to base any definitive conclusions about the behavioural effects of oral contraceptive agents.

Moos (10), using his Menstrual Distress Questionnaire, noted great variability in the individual response to oral contraceptives, which appeared to be greater in reaction to sequential than to combination preparations.

Kane *et al.* (6), in their numerous studies, have made a significant contribution to this area of investigation. They have reported changes in mood and behaviour in patients using progestational steroids for the treatment of severe pre-menstrual mood disturbances. Oral contraceptives were found to have a beneficial effect on the symptoms and mood of female psychiatric patients. Depression, irritability and lethargy occurred in some of these patients as well as in a non-psychiatric control group, but differences did not reach statistically significant levels. Their data reflected more perceived change of an unfavourable nature than had been reported previously and seemed to indicate increased risk of occurrence of such symptomatology in psychiatric patients. The changes, according to the authors, were very similar to those associated with the use of steroid hormones of many kinds. They found alterations in catecholmaine excretion associated with the use of oral contraceptives, which may lead to emotional disturbance, especially affective disorders.

154

Careful double blind placebo studies of effects over an extended period of time are needed in order to separate the drug effect from the issue of contraception.

Nilsson (11) and co-workers, in a retrospective study of the psychiatric changes associated with the use of an oral contraceptive, reported an increase in psychiatric symptoms in 17 per cent of their patients. Analysis of the material revealed, among many items recorded, depressive symptoms, impaired sexual adaptation (essentially decreased libido) and weight increase. The authors stated that the possibility of a causal connection between oral contraceptives and the mental symptoms should engage the attention of the clinician. In addition, favourable effects on premenstrual tension and dysmenorrhea were reported, as well as improvement in sexual adjustment for 50 per cent of the women.

Ruth Lidz (8) in her perceptive article discussed the role of emotional factors in the success of contraception and suggested guidelines for the success or failure of contraceptive medication. Based on a careful study of a small series of cases, she concluded that decrease of libido and depression in response to the pill were psychological reactions due to conflict over accepting or not accepting the contraceptive effect.

Grounds et al (3)† reported data from a double blind controlled comparison of the effects of a contraceptive and an inert pill. They correlated side effects with questionnaire-assessed neuroticism. Women on the active pill reported significantly more symptoms which decreased on the second month of the comparative study. No relationship was found between the presence of these symptoms and the degree of neuroticism in patients on the active pill.

Herzberg and Coppen (4)† selected 152 women at a family planning clinic near London who were about to use the pill for the first time and by way of control these women were compared with forty women attending the same clinic and about to commence using other contraceptive methods. A questionnaire concerning menstrual symptoms was administered, and the results agreed with Nilsson's — that the medication relieved dysmenorrhea in the majority of cases. A statistically significant number of women on the pill developed psychological side effects, including depression, and those who experienced depressive spells had higher neuroticism and extraversion scores.

Method

This study was based on a cross-sectional and longitudinal examination of seventy women attending either a gynæcologist in his private practice or a community family planning clinic. The co-operation of these non-psychiatric subjects was arranged by the referring physician. Women with organic gynæcological illness or with a history of psychiatric illness were excluded. Proven fertility and the use of medication for at least three months were conditional criteria for inclusion. Pills of different composition were administered, including both combination and sequential preparations, and the results reported do not relate to any specific compound.

Each of these women was interviewed in semi-structured and partly open interviews which lasted for several hours, permitting access to preconscious material. Regular follow-up interviews over a period of several months were arranged. Almost without exception these women readily co-operated; they welcomed the opportunity to vent their anxieties and to unburden themselves.

No control group was used; each woman in view of her previous history served as her own control.

On the strength of the interview material each of the women examined was subjected to a personality assessment according to the methods used by Jahoda (5) and Ruesch (12) in their classical studies. Each of the two interviewers (J.P. and L.T.) gave a personality rating at the end of the interview, after which two other psychiatrists (J.N.F. and E.D.W.) repeated the rating independently on the basis of the collated clinical material. When discrepancies oc-

†References 3 and 4 pertain to findings which appeared while our data were in the process of analysis.

curred the divergences of opinion were discussed until agreement could be reached.

The initial rating scale had three categories: A) no emotional maladjustment; B) minor emotional maladjustment with transient symptoms; and C) moderate emotional maladjustment. Clinical judgment and assessment of the subjects permitted a subdivision of the median group B into reactive and personality disorders, using a model from epidemiological research (7). In the final analysis the research was confined to two groups, A and C, adding reactive personality disorders to group A and minor personality disorders to group C. As stated before, women with gross psychiatric disorders were excluded from this series.

As regards physical and psychological side effects of the anovulants, a list of items was prepared with the aid of our gynæcological colleagues. This list was covered by the interviewers in each interview.

Other variables considered were: previous contraceptive methods, if any; reasons for change to oral contraceptives; symptoms during previous pregnancies; attitude of the husband toward contraception and oral contraceptives; current marital interaction; sexual compatibility, and financial situation.

Whenever possible, these items and variables were rated on a a scale ranging from one to four; also whenever possible they were correlated with the personality assessment (see above).

Findings

Onset of side effects. In some of the subjects 'side effects' appeared shortly after starting oral contraceptives, sometimes after a few days or weeks of medication. Because these early manifestations often subsided or disappeared afterwards it appeared unlikely that they were due to œstrogen effects, and more probable that they were due to fear and anticipation of ill effects.

The association of fears and anticipation of ill effects with their early appearance reached a statistical significance ($p<0.01$). Such fears, fostered by mass media, are common. Prominent among them were fears of cancer and of pregnancy despite the pill.

Less common was the fear of having malformed children on cessation of the medication and the fear of doing permanent damage to the procreative system. The repeatedly made statement: 'It can't be natural, one shouldn't tamper with things that should be left alone', not only indicates such fear but also a hidden regret for not having another baby. A woman who is afraid of having side effects from taking oral contraceptives is likely to have transient disturbing sensations or manifestations.

Nature of side effects. A multitude of somatic and psychological side effects was noted in our series. Very commonly reported at the somatic level were nausea, vomiting, swelling of the breasts and weight gain, and at the psychological level changes in mood and decline in libidinal interest. Common in the somatic sphere were gastrointestinal complaints such as disturbances of appetite and stomach pains and in the psychological sphere anxiety, irritability and nervousness. Uncommonly reported side effects were dizziness, headache and breakthrough bleeding.

Correlation of frequency and severity of side effects with personality assessment. Should it be true that side effects of oral contraceptive medication be to some extent or largely due to emotional factors it could be assumed that emotionally-maladjusted women have more severe side effects than emotionally well-adjusted women. With this hypothesis in mind the women in this series were divided according to their personality adjustment into those regarded as well-adjusted and those regarded as maladjusted and, according to the severity of side effects manifested, into those with no or minimal side effects and those with mild or moderate side effects (See Table I).

Correlation of the two sets of variables showed that the better emotionally adjusted a woman is the less likely she is to have side effects from taking oral contraceptives, that emotional adjustment did not exempt a woman from having mild or moderate side effects and that minor side effects quite commonly occurred in women rated as

TABLE I
DEGREE OF SIDE EFFECTS IN RELATION WITH PERSONALITY

Degree of side effects	Personality		Total
	N – 40 Well-adjusted	N – 30 Maladjusted	
Grade I or II (None or minimal)	33	14	47
Grade III or IV (Mild to moderate)	7	16	23
			70

LEGEND:
Personality Groups
Well-adjusted: No emotional maladjustment and/or minor reaction to environmental stress.
Maladjusted: Personality disorder and/or evidence of moderate emotional maladjustment.
Degree of Side Effects:
Group I – No side effects.
Group II – A minimum of physical and/or psychological side effects such as fullness of breasts and weight gain.
Group III – A cluster of physiological and/or psychological side effects which are felt as mildly disturbing and interfere with the woman's functioning to a minor degree.
Group IV – A cluster of physiological and/or psychological side effects which moderately or severely disturb or incapacitate the woman.

emotionally maladjusted. This statement should not be misunderstood as meaning that all side effects are due to emotional factors. Such an assumption would be clearly absurd as regards such side effects as fullness of breasts, weight gain and some of the menstrual disturbances.

Correlation of the nature of side effects with personality assessment. Some of these side effects such as weight gain and swelling of the breasts seem to be biological in origin and others such as depression, irritability and decline in libidinal interest seem to be psychological in origin, while still others such as fatigue, nausea and vomiting may have been of both or either origin. Should this be true it would be expected that there would be an accumulation of psychological side effects in emotionally-maladjusted women, no correlation between biological side effects with either emotional adjustment or maladjustment and differential results regarding side effects thought to be of doubtful origin.

This hypothesis was confirmed, in that it was found that depressive symptomatology and decline in libidinal interest on oral con-

traceptive medication were significantly correlated with emotional maladjustment; that no such correlation existed between weight gain and emotional maladjustment; and that nausea and vomiting were associated with emotional maladjustment while fatigue was not.

Puzzling and unaccountable is the statistically significant association of breast engorgement as a side effect of the pill with emotional maladjustment (See Tables II and III).

Depression and decline of libidinal interest. These two side effects deserve special attention:

a) *Depression*: 45 per cent of the women studied displayed depressive symptomatology while on oral contraceptive medication. They felt unhappy and dejected, lost appetite, weight and sexual interest, cried a great deal, had self-accusatory ideas and some of them had suicidal ruminations.

Some of these women had had depressive states long before they started on the drug, and these continued, improved or became worse without any demonstrable connection with the medication. During the many years

157

TABLE II
NAUSEA AND/OR VOMITING IN RELATION TO PERSONALITY

Nausea and/or vomiting	Personality		
	A = 40	C = 30	
Present	6	11	17
Absent	34	19	53
			70

X2 : 4.3766 X^2_c : 3.2776 $p < 0.10$.

of medication others had had depressive reactions which were apparently unrelated to the drug but were in response to environmental stress, as in the case of the woman whose grief over her father's death passed into a state of melancholia. But there remains still another group of women whose depressive symptoms started shortly after being placed on the oral contraceptive pill, continued during this medication but lifted when taken off the pill and especially after becoming pregnant.

While the possibility may not be excluded that in these cases the depressive spell was due to alteration in the hormonal system, a psychological explanation can also be offered. Careful study of the case histories shows that this type of reaction occurred in women who, forced by circumstances, reluctantly agreed to take the pill. There is therefore good reason to believe that the limitation of the depressive symptomatology

to the period of oral contraceptive medication is not due to the drug but to a conflict between the professed desire for birth control and an unrecognized desire for more children.

b) *Decline in libidinal interests*: because fear of a further pregnancy was the main reason for taking oral contraceptives in the women in this series, it was assumed that the safety of the pill, as compared with other contraceptive measures, would increase their libidinal interest and their pleasure in sexual intercourse. However, this proved true for only slightly over 35 per cent of the sample. In the remainder, libidinal interest either remained unchanged or decreased (See Table IV).

Prominent among those whose libidinal interest remained unchanged were women who failed to trust the effectiveness of the pill, that is, those in whom the fear-alleviating effect of taking it did not materialize,

TABLE III
BREAST ENGORGEMENT IN RELATION TO PERSONALITY

Breast engorgement	Personality		
	A = 40	C = 30	
Present	11	16	27
Absent	29	14	43
			70

X2 = 4.8284 X^2_c = 3.7997 $p < 0.10$.

TABLE IV
SEXUAL INTEREST IN RELATION TO PERSONALITY

Sexual interest (Libido)	Personality		
	A = 40	C = 30	
Improved	20	7	27
Unchanged	14	9	23
Decreased	6	14	20
			70

$X^2 = 9.3076$ $p < 0.01$.

and also among those who had been frigid previously. A woman who is frigid is not likely to be less frigid because she takes the pill.

As regards decline in libidinal interest three factors, in isolation or in combination, contributed to it: previous emotional maladjustment, previous sexual maladjustment and marital discord. In this respect two constellations were commonly encountered, one related to reduction in restraint in sexual activities and the other, strangely enough, related to the effectiveness of the pill as a contraceptive agent. Typical of the former constellation is the story of an anxious, irritable, ill-tempered neurotic woman whose relationship with her husband had been strained for years. After the birth of three children the husband and wife decided to have no more and she began taking contraceptive medication. She had never been 'keen on sex' or at least was less keen than her husband. With having no excuse for the wife to refuse herself, quarrels ensued, with the result that the misery of the marriage and concomitantly her aversion to sexual intercourse increased. Typical of the latter situation is the woman who after the birth of two children had bowed to the financial necessity to have no more. She had asked for an effective contraceptive method but in the deep layers of her mind (and perhaps not even so unconsciously) she longed for more children. In response to her sense of frustration she passed into a state of de-

pression with concomitant decrease in sexual interest.

Summary and Conclusion

It has been shown that physcial and psychological manifestations appearing very early after the commencement of oral contraceptive medication can hardly be attributed to œstrogen effects, but are more likely to be due to fear and the anticipation of ill effects. Of the multitude of physical and psychological manifestations complained of by women on the drug some are of somatic origin and others of psychological origin, and women who are emotionally well-adjusted are less likely to report side effects than those who are emotionally maladjusted. Some reasons for depressive spells and for decline in libidinal interest on oral contraceptive medication have been discussed. One factor which emerged is that some women who ask for safe contraceptives, in fact hanker for pregnancy and childbirth, while contraception signifies prevention of impregnation for the time being — temporary infertility. Infertility however temporary and however planned and the unwarranted dread of permanent infertility have a profound emotionally disturbing effect on many women.

The results obtained should be considered with due regard for possible methodological errors. For instance it might be objected that no control group was used, but to find a control group for studies of this kind is

159

difficult and to use women on a placebo as controls is obviously out of the question. The general validity of the observation may be limited because the women in this study were either Jewish or Anglo-Protestants. Differences might have been seen had members of other ethnic or religious groups been studied. The retrospective nature of the investigation might imply some distortions, but the use of semi-structured interviews with specific items on a ranging scale partially obviated the possible impressionistic quality of the material. The 'halo effect' which occurs in a personal interview was corrected by the introduction of multi-raters and the experienced clinical judgment of the investigators.

At the outset the intention was to find out which side effects of anovulants are biological in origin and which are psychological. This objective has been accomplished to some extent, but more important perhaps are the practical implications of the research. On the strength of these observations a gynæcologist or a family physician may be well-advised to listen with the 'third ear' to a woman who consults him, in order to make sure that she really wants a safe contraceptive and not a baby. Undue anxiety regarding the ill effects of the pill, fostered by alarming reports spread by the mass media, should be dispelled. Before prescribing the pill, evidence of emotional maladjustment in the woman or problems in her marriage (sexual or other) should be looked for. The physician should also look for reasons for depression and for decline in libidinal interest in the woman when placed on contraceptive medication. In others words, he should concern himself with the personality of his patient, rather than confining himself to her biological functions.

Acknowledgements

This study was made possible with the financial assistance of G. D. Searle through the Medical Director, Dr. H. R. Hutchings. The investigation was continued with the help of the Federal-Provincial Mental Health Project 604-7-651. We wish to acknowledge their help and express our gratitude for their assistance.

We also wish to express our thanks to the many colleagues who have collaborated in this investigation; especially to Dr. M. Bérard, Head of Gynaecology and Obstetrics, Université de Montréal and Dr. Y. Lefebvre at Hôpital Notre Dame, also to Dr. M. M. Gelfand, Head of the Department of Gynaecology at the Jewish General Hospital who made this research possible by referring many private patients, and to Dr. R. Kinch, Head of Gynaecology at the Montreal General Hospital who was instrumental in facilitating access to the clinic patients. We also thank Mrs. Francie Piva for her loyalty, patience and diligent secretarial work.

References

1. Bakker, C. B., Dightman, C. R.: Side effects of oral contraceptives, *Obstet. Gynec.,* 28, 373-379, 1966.
2. Glick, I. A.: Mood and behavioural changes associated with the use of oral contraceptive agents, *Psychopharmacologia (Berl.)* VJ, 363-374, 1967.
3. Grounds, D., et al.: The contraceptive pill, side effects and personality: Report of a controlled double blind trial, *Brit. J. Psychiat.,* 116, 169-172, 1970.
4. Herzberg, B., Coppen, A.: Changes in psychologic symptoms in women taking oral contraceptives, *Brit. J. Psychiat.,* 116, 161-164, 1970.
5. Jahoda, M.: "Current Concepts of Positive Mental Health" in *Joint Commission on Mental Illness and Health"*, Monograph 1, New York, Basic Books, 1958.
6. Kane, F. et al.: Emotional change associated with oral contraceptives in female psychiatric patients, *Comprehensive Psychiatry,* 10, 16-30, 1969.
7. Leighton, A. H., et al.: Validity in mental health surveys, *Canad. Psychiat. Ass. J.,* 11, 167-178, 1966.
8. Lidz, Ruth: Emotional factors in the success of contraception, *Fertil. and Steril.,* 20, 761-771, 1969.
9. Lipowski, Z. J.: New perspectives in psychosomatic medicine, *Canad. Psychiat. Ass. J.,* 15, 515-525, 1970.
10. Moos, R.: Psychological aspects of oral contraceptives, *Arch. Gen. Psychiat.,* 19, 87-94, 1968.
11. Nilsson, A., et al.: Side effects of an oral contraceptive with particular attention to mental symptoms and sexual adaptation, *Acta Obst. Gynec. Scand.,* 46, 537-556, 1967.
12. Ruesch, J.: The infantile personality, *Psychosom. Med.,* 10, 134-144, 1948.

INFLUENCE OF CONTRACEPTIVE GESTOGEN PILLS ON SEXUAL BEHAVIOUR AND THE SPREAD OF GONORRHOEA

BY

LENNART JUHLIN AND STURE LIDÉN

The introduction and widespread use of antibiotics in the last few decades have altered public attitudes towards venereal diseases and the previous fear of their consequences has been replaced by indifference, which has in turn contributed to sexual permissiveness. It has been contended that the removal of fear of pregnancy by the increasing availability and use of contraceptive gestogen pills and intrauterine devices has also contributed to increased sexual activity and has thus possibly become a new factor facilitating the spread of venereal infections (Idsøe and Guthe, 1967).

The use of contraceptive gestogen pills has increased in Sweden during the last two years and the present study was undertaken to obtain answers to the following questions:

(1) Does the use of gestogen contraceptive pills lead to an increase of promiscuous behaviour?

(2) What is the effect of such pills on the frequency of sexual intercourse?

(3) Is there evidence that such hormonal ingestion alters the susceptibility of the mucosa to gonococcal infection?

(4) Has the use of condoms—so far considered the best protection against venereal diseases—decreased since the introduction of the gestogen pills?

Material and Methods

Patients

The Venereal Disease Clinic of the University Hospital, Uppsala, serves an area of approximately 100,000 people, of whom 19,000 (19 per cent.) were registered as university students at the time of the present study. The investigation involved a total of 522 patients who attended this venereal disease outpatients clinic from September, 1967, to February, 1968. Among these 522 patients, 250 (47·8 per cent.) were

females and 272 (52·2 per cent.) males. Of the total patients of both sexes, 182 (34·8 per cent.) were university students. Among the 250 females there were 71 (28·4 per cent.) university students and among the 272 males there were 111 (40·7 per cent.). These categories and the age and sex distribution of the study group are contained in Table I.

TABLE I
CATEGORY, AGE, AND SEX DISTRIBUTION OF PATIENTS

Sex	Category	< 20 yrs	20–25 yrs	> 25 yrs	Total
Male	University students	4	86	21	111
	Non-students	27	79	55	161
Female	University students	6	57	8	71
	Non-students	73	80	26	179
Total		110	302	110	522

A clinical diagnosis of gonorrhoea was confirmed by positive cultures in 147 (54 per cent.) of the males and 168 (67 per cent.) of the females. The patients in whom gonorrhoea was not diagnosed by these criteria had been named as contacts of patients with proven gonorrhoea. In accordance with the venereal disease legislation in force in Sweden at the time of the study, these sexual partners are obliged to undergo medical examination.

Method of Survey

All patients were informed that factors which might contribute to the spread of gonorrhoea were being investigated. They were asked if they would participate in an investigation and give honest replies to intimate questions, and all except three replied to the questions posed orally by the special interviewer. The replies were recorded in a questionnaire. To prevent misunderstanding, all questions were carefully explained. The patients were asked to write down the number of their sexual partners during the last year and the number

161

of days per month they estimated that they had sexual intercourse. It was explained that it was important to know how much time had elapsed before they suspected they had been exposed to gonorrhoea. An affirmative in reply to the question whether male partners always or nearly always used condoms was recorded as "yes"; "no" meant that they rarely or never used condoms. When completed the questionnaire was deposited by the patient through a slot into a sealed box.

Results

These are presented in Tables II to VI.

(1) Of the different contraceptives, oral gestogen pills were predominant among females examined. They were used by 70·4 per cent. of the students and 50·1 per cent. of the non-student patients (Table II). Among the latter, gestogen pills were used by 36 per cent. of those under 20 years of age and by 63 per cent. of those between 20 and 25 years. Diaphragms were used by eight patients and intrauterine loops by two patients in both groups together.

TABLE II

STUDENTS AND NON-STUDENTS USING CONTRACEPTIVES

Type of Contraceptive	Students		Non-students	
	No.	Per cent.	No.	Per cent.
Pills	50	70·4	91	50·1
Diaphragm	6	8·4	2	1·1
Intrauterine loop	0	0	2	1·1
Condom	40	36·0	40	24·3

(2) Patients less than 20 years of age had more partners than those over 25 years (Table III).

TABLE III

FREQUENCY OF INTERCOURSE PER MONTH AND NUMBER OF PARTNERS PER YEAR OF PATIENTS USING AND NOT USING CONTRACEPTIVE PILLS. MEAN ±SE

Pills	Age (yrs)	No. of Women	Frequency of Intercourse	No. of Partners
Taken	< 20	31	7·2±1·0	3·7±0·5
	20–25	91	7·5±0·5**	3·4±0·3*
	> 25	19	6·1±1·6	2·4±0·4
Not taken	< 20	48	5·7±0·9	3·3±0·3
	20–25	46	5·1±0·9	2·5±0·2
	> 25	15	5·9±2·0	2·0±0·3

*P < 0·05.
**P < 0·01.
P—The probability that the difference between patients with and without pills is caused by random factors

Patients between 20 and 25 years taking gestogen pills had 36 per cent. more sexual partners than those of the same age not taking pills (P<0·05);

20 per cent. of all women taking pills had more than ten partners per year and 26 per cent. one partner. The same percentages were found among those not taking pills. Among the patients having two to ten partners, the mean number of such partners was probably higher in those using pills than in those not using them (P<0·05).

The frequency of sexual intercourse per month was about 47 per cent. higher among patients aged 20–25 years taking pills (P<0·01; Table III). The patients' replies to the question whether the number of partners or the frequency of sexual intercourse had increased after they started using pills are shown in Table IV. Although most patients believed that their sexual activities had not changed significantly, there was an increase rather than decrease in the number of partners and in the frequency of intercourse after they had started using gestogen pills (P<0·01). About one-fifth of the patients were unable to reply to these questions, mainly because of irregular sexual activity.

TABLE IV

NUMBER OF PATIENTS DECLARING A CHANGE IN FREQUENCY OF SEXUAL INTERCOURSE AND NUMBER OF PARTNERS AFTER COMMENCING TO USE CONTRACEPTIVE GESTOGEN PILLS

Frequency of Intercourse	No. of Patients Stating Frequency of Intercourse	Patients stating No. of Partners
Increased	43	25
Decreased	9	10
Unchanged	63	84

(3) A diagnosis of gonorrhoea was made as frequently among those using pills as among those not using them (Table V). A history of previous gonococcal infection was noted in 12 per cent. of the female university students and 30 per cent. of the non-students. There was no difference in the percentage of previous infection in the women taking pills compared to those not taking pills.

TABLE V

PATIENTS WITH POSITIVE GONOCOCCAL CULTURES AMONG THOSE USING AND NOT USING CONTRACEPTIVE GESTOGEN PILLS

Pills	University students		Non-students		Total	
	Per cent.	No.	Per cent.	No.	Per cent.	No.
Taken	52	26	77	70	68	96
Not taken	52	11	69	61	66	72

(4) Of male student patients 36 per cent. and of the male non-student patients 24·3 per cent. used condoms; 40 per cent. of those below 20 years

of age used condoms. Patients having more than ten partners per year used condoms to the same extent as those with only one to three partners (Table VI). This Table also shows that the use of condoms was about twice as frequent among those having intercourse only once per month as among those having intercourse on more than ten occasions.

TABLE VI

PERCENTAGE OF PATIENTS USING CONDOMS
ACCORDING TO NUMBER OF PARTNERS AND
FREQUENCY OF INTERCOURSE

Number of Partners per Year				Monthly Frequency of Intercourse			
1	2–3	4–10	10	1	2–4	5–10	10
25	25	36	28	42	32	29	20

Four non-student females using gestogen pills stated that their partners used condoms. Among those not taking pills the partner used condoms in 71 per cent. of the university students and 27 per cent. of the others.

Discussion

Though the majority of female patients declared that there had been no change in the number of partners after starting to use contraceptive pills, 25 stated that the number of partners had increased whereas only ten had a decreased number of partners after starting to take pills. When the mean number of partners of all patients between 20 and 25 years of age was estimated, an increase of 36 per cent. was found in the group using pills. The question whether the use of pills gives rise to increased promiscuity must therefore be answered in the affirmative. It is likely that this may contribute to an increased spread of gonorrhoea. An increased number of partners was more frequent among young people and a shift of gonorrhoea to younger ages will thus also increase its spread. This makes it difficult to evaluate the importance of the increased number of partners associated with the use of pills. We investigated pill usage in a similar group of women attending the clinic in 1966 (Juhlin, 1968), and since that time it has increased from 23 to 56 per cent. The age distribution is the same, but the number of patients with gonorrhoea treated in the clinic has increased by 10 per cent. This figure depends, however, on many factors and cannot be analysed further on the basis of the present data.

As regards the effect of oral contraceptives on the frequency of intercourse, we found that they increased the frequency by about 25 per cent. in the student and non-student group as a whole. The

probable reason for this is the feeling of safety from conception when using contraceptive pills; it does not necessarily mean that the pills cause increase in libido. Reports in the literature on the effect of the pills on libido as such are divergent (Drill, 1966; Larsson-Cohn, 1966), both increase and decrease having been reported. Enjoyment of sexual intercourse is often found to be increased (Larsson-Cohn, 1966, Nilsson, Jacobson, and Ingemanson, 1967) or not affected (Nilsson and Sölvell, 1967).

Although oral gestogen pills may be held to increase the susceptibility of the mucosa to gono-coccal infection, we found no evidence of this, since gonorrhoea was diagnosed to the same extent among those taking pills as among the controls. Since the women not using pills more often had partners using condoms than those using pills, this should have tended to decrease the frequency of gonorrhoea in this group. The absence of such a decrease may be due to the fact that the partners only used condoms on certain occasions as a contraceptive and even then not during the entire intercourse in an attempt to prevent venereal disease. If condoms had been used regularly and during the entire exposure time, the partners would have been unlikely to have acquired gonorrhoea. The possibility also exists that the pills decrease the susceptibility of the mucosa to gonorrhoea.

It should be pointed out that a similar incidence of gonorrhoea among those using and not using gestogen pills does not mean that their use has no effect on the spread of gonorrhoea. The increased sexual activity among patients taking pills probably increases their proportion in clinic patients.

On investigating the use of contraceptives by the patients attending the clinic in 1966, we found that 18 per cent. of the non-students and 48 per cent. of the University students used pills. In 1968, the total percentage of patients using pills was more than doubled. The increased use of pills was not, however, accompanied by a decreased use of condoms, which were still used by about one-third of the men. This is the same figure as was found previously. Only four of the patients taking pills had partners using condoms. In the earlier investigation 54 per cent. of the women said that one of the partners used a contraceptive. This figure is now increased to 73 per cent. due to increased use of contraceptive pills.

Summary

The influence of the use of contraceptive gestogen pills on human sexual behaviour and on the possible spread of gonorrhoea was investigated among 522 patients attending the Venereal Disease Clinic in Uppsala, Sweden, from September 1967, to February, 1968. Among the 250 women, 71 (28·4 per cent.) were university students, and fifty of these (70·4 per cent.) used contraceptive pills. Among 179 non-student female patients, 91 (50·1 per cent.) used contraceptive pills. In 1966—about a year before the present study—the corresponding findings were 48 and 18 per cent. respectively. This considerable increase in the use of contraceptive pills was not accompanied by a decrease in the use of condoms, which were used by 30 per cent. of the men, as in 1966.

The number of sexual partners per year and the frequency of intercourse were significantly higher in the women taking pills than in the others, and were highest in the age group 20 to 25 years. In the whole study group more persons stated that the number of partners and the frequency of sexual intercourse had increased after starting to use contraceptive pills. It is considered that this increase in sexual activity probably increases the risk of gonococcal infection. Gonorrhoea was diagnosed in 67 per cent of the women. The remainder investigated were named as partners of patients with diagnosed disease. A diagnosis of gonorrhoea was made as frequently among those using pills as among those who did not. There is thus no evidence that the susceptibility of the mucosa to gonococcal infection is increased by the use of contraceptive gestogen pills.

The authors wish to thank Dr. Barbro Lewin and Miss Barbro Westrin for carefully interviewing the patients.
This study was supported by the Swedish Medical Research Council (Project No. B68-19X-769-03).

REFERENCES

DRILL, V. A. (1966). "Oral Contraceptives", p. 110–111. McGraw-Hill, New York.
IDSØE, O., and GUTHE, T. (1967). *Brit. J. vener. Dis.*, **43**, 227.
JUHLIN, L. (1968). *Acta derm.-venereol. (Stockh.)*, **48**, 82.

LARSSON-COHN, U. (1966). *Acta obstet. gynec. scand.*, **45**, 499.
NILSSON, Å., JACOBSON, L., and INGEMANSON, C. A. (1967). *Ibid.*, **46**, 537.
NILSSON, L., and SÖLVELL, L. (1967). *Ibid.*, **46**, Suppl. 8, "Studies on Oral Contraceptives".

INDIVIDUAL ASPIRATIONS AS RELATED TO EARLY AND LATE ACCEPTANCE OF CONTRACEPTION

S. B. KAR

A. INTRODUCTION

Literature suggests that probably the most significant determinant of the acceptance of contraception is neither the innovation of modern birth control methods nor the proselytizing efforts by various family planning organizations, but the initiative of individuals to control their own fertility (3, p. 67; 4, p. 78; 5, p. 2; 6, p. 3; 12, p. 1326; 18, pp. 34-35; 19, p. 20). This suggests the need to explore what motivates the eligible couples to accept contraception. But, so far, very little effort has been made to explore the motivational and social-psychological correlates of contraception. A bibliography of studies in fertility control edited by Tietze (23) indicates that, of a total of 1935 publications included, less than two percent dealt with the social-psychological and motivational dimensions of contraception.

The relationship between contraception and various demographic and socio-economic variables has been frequently investigated (5, 6, 11, 13, 18, 23, 24). Further research in these areas, though useful, may be less productive in bringing out new information as compared to research efforts in the area of social-psychological and motivational dimensions of contraception. This study is an attempt to explore the motivational correlates of contraception, with special reference to early and late acceptance of contraception.

1. Earlier Psychological Studies

The two major studies which have explored the social-psychological and personality dynamics of contraception (11, 24) have yielded negative results. Both studies used the outcome of behavior (size of planned family and fertility planning success), rather than contraception, as their dependent variable. At the time these studies were conducted, the failure of contraception was rather high due to lack of dependable methods (5, p. 209). Consequently, success or failure of contraception may not represent the extent of contraceptive practices by the couples nor the underlying psychological state related to contraception. In addition, the independent variables used in these studies are very broad and generalized psychological attributes. Such variables are not always helpful in predicting specific behavior. The selection of dependent and independent variables was probably largely responsible for the inconclusive findings of these studies.

2. *Conceptual Framework of this Study*

This study attempts to explore the motivational patterns associated with contraception, especially early and late acceptance of contraception. Since one behavior may be determined by multiple motives, it is assumed that the motivational correlates of contraception should be studied through a holistic and subjective frame-of-reference. It is further assumed that a motivated behavior is influenced by the subjects' future orientation, social optimism, value orientations, and areas of satisfaction in life. This study thus tests five hypotheses:

Hypothesis I: There will be a significant and positive relationship between the level of striving and contraception.

Hypothesis II: There will be a significant and positive relationship between future orientation and contraception.

Hypothesis III: There will be a significant and positive relationship between value orientations and contraception.

Hypothesis IV: There will be a significant and positive relationship between social optimism and contraception.

Hypothesis V: There will be a significant and positive relationship between areas of satisfaction in life and contraception.

B. Method

1. *The Sample*

The sample consisted of 209 (white = 169, and nonwhite = 40) married women of lower socioeconomic status, in Berkeley, California. All subjects were living with their husbands and had at least one living child. The 1960 United States Housing Census data were used to select the census tracts with average value of owner-occupied houses and monthly rent less than the respective averages for entire Berkeley. A probability sample was drawn from a list of 1866 two-parent families obtained from four schools situated in school districts roughly corresponding to the selected census tracts with lower socioeconomic status. The nonresponse rate was about three percent.

2. *Definitions of Variables and Instrument of Data Collection*

Level of Striving (LOS) is defined as the degree of difficulty or proximity of an individual's action goals to his ideal goals (1, p. 22; 16, p. 81; 17,

p. 335). Striving is directed towards a subjective *Goal Constellation* which is defined in this study as subjective hopes, wishes, and desires on one end; and fears, worries, and concerns on the other end of an individual's self-anchoring continuum (1, p. 22). Cantril's Self-Anchoring Striving Scale (1, 2), was used to obtain data on goal-constellation and level of striving. An additional item was introduced in this scale to obtain subjective ranking of the aspired goals. The scale measured level of striving (LOS) for three different time points: past LOS (five years ago), present LOS, and future LOS (five years hence).

Future Orientation (FO) is defined as an individual's willingness to sacrifice his short-term goals and day-to-day conveniences for long-term desirable goals (10, p. 124). Future Orientation was measured by means of a scale of eight paired-items, one item in each pair representing a relatively short-term goal as compared to the other (10, pp. 124-125). Each preference of a relatively long-term goal was scored as one, and short-term as zero.

Value Orientations (VO) are categorized under two classes: (*a*) activistic, individualistic, and future-time orientations as defined by Kluckhohn (14) and Rosen (20, 21) are classified as positive value orientations; and (*b*) passivistic, familistic, and present-time orientations are classified as negative value orientations. Value Orientations were measured by means of a six-item scale after Rosen's (20) value orientation scale. Each positive value oriented response was scored as one; other responses as zero.

Social Optimism (SO) is defined as an individual's belief that (*a*) social order is predictable, (*b*) social collaborators are trustworthy, (*c*) the future has potential for improvement, (*d*) community leadership is sympathetic to the common man's needs, and (*e*) it is worthwhile to sacrifice present pleasure for the sake of future. Srole's (22) anomie scale was used to measure social optimism. Each disagreement with the scale item was scored as one; other responses as zero.

Areas of Satisfaction in Life (ASL) is defined as subjective feeling of satisfaction in the following areas: (*a*) day-to-day needs and comforts, (*b*) short-term material goals, (*c*) long-term material goals, (*d*) education of children, (*e*) personal interests, and (*f*) old-age security. A six-item scale was constructed after Knutson's (15) scale of areas of satisfaction in life to measure subjective satisfaction in selected areas of life. Satisfaction in each area was scored as one, other responses as zero.

Socioeconomic Status (SES) is defined, after Hollingshead (7, 8, 9), in terms of husband's social position index on a two-factor social position scale. Hollingshead's (7, 8) two-factor index of social position was used to measure socioeconomic status. On each of these variables, the subjects scoring equal or above the median were placed in "high" category, while those scoring below the median were placed in the "low" category.

Contraception is defined as reported use of birth control methods for the purpose of spacing and/or regulating pregnancies. Use of birth control methods for other reasons is not considered as acceptance of contraception. Acceptors of contraception are those who were continuous users of birth control methods, and when they discontinued, it was because they wanted a child, were temporarily separated, or the wife was pregnant; but resumed use of birth control methods as soon as such conditions were over. Those who never used any method of birth control, were not sterile, and were either undecided or opposed to contraception were classified as nonacceptors. The remaining were defined as unclassified.

The subjective reporting method was used and the data were collected through individual interviews.

C. Results and Discussions

Of all subjects, about three percent were nonacceptors of contraception, and 16 percent were unclassified. The data suggest that contraception is significantly related to race and socioeconomic status. Sixty percent of the whites as against 31 percent of the nonwhites initially accepted contraception before the second pregnancy ($\chi^2 = 9.03$, $df = 1$, $p < .005$). Among the white subjects, 62 percent of the "high" SES group as against 37 percent of the "low" SES group were early acceptors ($\chi^2 = 17.68$, $df = 1$, $p < .001$). Among the whites, 45 percent accepted contraception before the first pregnancy, 17 percent after the first but before the second pregnancy, 26 percent after the second but before the fourth pregnancy, and the remaining 12 percent after the fourth pregnancy.

1. *Test of Hypotheses*

The hypotheses were tested by comparing 69 early and 86 late acceptors of contraception among the white subjects only. Since the numbers of nonwhites and nonacceptors were small, such subjects were excluded. The *early acceptors* were those who reportedly accepted contraception before the first pregnancy, and the *late acceptors* were those who reportedly accepted contraception after the first pregnancy. Each hypothesis was tested while socioeconomic status was held constant.

2. *Hypothesis I: Level of Striving and Contraception*

Although the early and the late acceptors aspired for similar goals, the subjective ranking of the nine categories of life-goals varied (tau $= .38$, $p >$

.05). The subjective life-goals were classified under nine categories of aspirations related to (a) children, (b) social status (improvement), (c) self-improvement, (d) health (self and family), (e) economic status maintenance, (f) long-term material goals, (g) short-term material goals, (h) close family relationship, and (i) peace and social order. The nine categories of life-goals were ranked according to how frequently each was placed within the three top positions by the subjects. The early acceptors more frequently than the late acceptors placed improvement of social status, self-improvement, and close family ties among the three top ranking goals. The late acceptors on the other hand, more frequently placed economic and material goals among the top three ranks. This suggests that the early acceptors were more frequently concerned with long-term and promotive goals.

The early and the late acceptors were more alike in their worries about the future (tau $= .86$, $p < .001$). Major worries were related to health, economic status, war or violence, and children.[1]

The data suggest that level of striving (LOS) is significantly and positively related with contraception, as well as with socioeconomic status (SES). The correlation coefficients between contraception and LOS are past LOS, $r = .44$; present LOS, $r = .58$; and future LOS, $r = .56$. The zero order correlation coefficients are significant at the .001 level. The subjects of "high" SES had significantly higher mean of present LOS scores than the subjects of "low" SES group ("high" SES: mean $= 6.89$, $SD = 1.52$; "low" SES: mean $= 5.71$, $SD = 1.81$; $t = 4.29$; $df = 153$; $p < .001$).

Table 1 shows the mean scores of LOS for three time points by early and late acceptance of contraception while SES is held constant.

Within each SES category, the mean LOS of the early acceptors is significantly higher than the mean LOS of the late acceptors. The difference of LOS between the early and the late acceptors is greater in the "low" SES than in the "high" SES (Table 1). This is probably because, in the upper social status, early acceptance of contraception has become a widely shared social norm. In the absence of such a norm in the lower social status, it is likely that a person needs greater individual initiative to accept contraception at the very early stage of his married life. Further analysis indicated that the early acceptors had significantly greater upward mobility of LOS than the late acceptors (mobility of LOS is the difference between past and present LOS; and present and future LOS).

---

[1] For Appendix items 1 through 5, order NAPS Document 01268 from CCM Information Corp. ——NAPS, 909 Third Avenue, New York, New York 10022, remitting $2.00 for microfiche or $5.00 for photocopies.

TABLE 1
MEAN SCORES OF LEVEL OF STRIVING (LOS) BY EARLY AND LATE ACCEPTANCE OF
CONTRACEPTION WITH SOCIOECONOMIC STATUS (SES) HELD CONSTANT

Level of striving	Early acceptors		Late acceptors		
	Mean	SD	Mean	SD	t
Present LOS					
All SES	6.83	1.39	5.50	1.57	5.51**
High SES	7.00	1.21	6.14	1.71	2.01*
Low SES	6.48	1.81	5.00	1.23	4.21**
Past LOS					
All SES	4.80	1.73	3.70	1.82	3.12**
High SES	4.57	1.34	3.71	2.16	1.87*
Low SES	4.30	2.34	3.21	1.40	2.58*
Future LOS					
All SES	8.35	.87	7.58	1.14	4.62**
High SES	8.96	.84	8.25	1.04	2.91**
Low SES	8.43	.95	7.26	1.05	4.62**

Note: df: all SES = 153, high SES = 72, low SES = 79.
** $p < .01$.
* $p < .05$.

The data indicate that level of striving is significantly and positively related to early acceptance of contraception. The patterns of life-goals of the early and the late acceptors also varied. It is thus likely that both the goals a person aspires for and his level of striving may determine how early he will accept contraception.

3. Hypothesis II: Future Orientation and Contraception

Future orientation (FO) is significantly and positively related with contraception, as well as with SES. While nearly two-thirds of the early acceptors scored "high" in future orientation (equal or above median), nearly 60 percent of the late acceptors scored "low" ($\chi^2 = 8.17$, $df = 1$, $p < .005$). The mean FO scores for the "high" SES group (5.62, $SD = 1.61$) was significantly higher than the corresponding mean for the "low" SES group (4.80, $SD = 2.22$; $t = 7.74$; $df = 153$; $p < .001$).

Table 2.1 shows the mean FO scores by early and late acceptance of contraception while SES is held constant. Although FO is positively related with SES, when SES is held constant the mean FO scores of the early acceptors is significantly higher than the corresponding mean of the late acceptors (Table 2.I) within each SES subgroup.[2]

---

2 See footnote 1.

TABLE 2
MEAN SCORES OF FUTURE ORIENTATION, VALUE ORIENTATIONS, SOCIAL OPTIMISM, AND AREAS OF SATISFACTION IN LIFE BY EARLY AND LATE ACCEPTANCE OF CONTRACEPTION WITH *SES* HELD CONSTANT

Psychological variables	Early acceptors Mean	SD	Late acceptors Mean	SD	t
I. Future Orientation					
All SES	5.69	1.55	4.38	2.15	4.41**
High SES	5.89	1.50	4.98	1.76	2.33*
Low SES	5.83	1.80	4.40	2.18	3.06**
II. Value Orientations					
All SES	4.62	1.90	3.91	1.44	2.73**
High SES	5.13	.72	4.01	.82	5.66**
Low SES	4.12	.67	3.47	1.06	2.33*
III. Social Optimism					
All SES	3.78	1.25	1.98	1.36	3.76**
High SES	4.09	1.03	3.47	1.07	2.08*
Low SES	3.17	1.44	2.59	1.40	2.31*
IV. Areas of Satisfaction					
All SES	3.72	1.47	3.47	1.59	1.01ns
High SES	3.78	1.26	4.00	1.52	.68ns
Low SES	3.61	1.85	3.21	1.58	1.00ns

Note: SES = socioeconomic status, ns = not significant at .05 level.
** $p < .01$.
* $p < .05$.

4. Hypothesis III: Value Orientations and Contraception

Value Orientations (VO) are significantly and positively related with contraception, as well as with SES. A significantly higher proportion of the early acceptors (60.8 percent) than the late acceptors (38.4 percent) obtained "high" VO scores ($\chi^2 = 7.91$; $df = 1$, $p < .005$). The mean VO score of the subjects of "high" SES (4.66; $SD = .78$) was significantly higher than the corresponding mean of the subjects of "low" SES (3.64, $SD = .91$, $t = 7.71$, $df = 153$, $p < .001$).

Table 2.II shows the mean VO scores by early and late acceptance of contraception while SES is held constant. Although VO is positively related with SES, when SES is held constant, the mean VO scores of the early acceptors is significantly higher than the corresponding mean of the late acceptors within each SES subgroup (Table 2.II). This suggests that positive value orientations are significantly and positively related with early acceptance of contraception regardless of the SES of the subjects.[3]

---

[3] See footnote 1.

5. *Hypothesis IV: Social Optimism and Contraception*

Social Optimism (SO) is significantly and positively related with contraception, as well as with SES. The proportion of subjects scoring "low" (less than median) on social optimism was significantly greater among the late acceptors (60.4 percent) than that among the early acceptors (37.65 percent; $\chi^2 = 7.94$, $df = 1$, $p < .005$). The mean SO scores of the subjects of "high" SES (3.89, $SD = 1.76$) was significantly higher than the corresponding mean of the subjects of "low" SES (2.83, $SD = 1.42$, $t = 5.30$, $df = 153$, $p < .001$).

Table 2.III shows the mean SO scores of the early and late acceptors while SES is held constant. Although SO is significantly and positively related with SES, when SES is held constant, the mean SO scores of the early acceptors is significantly higher than the corresponding mean of the late acceptors of contraception (Table 2.III). This suggests that social optimism is significantly and positively related with early acceptance of contraception regardless of the SES of the subjects. The data indicated that, as compared to the late acceptors, the early acceptors more frequently felt that their social collaborators are trustworthy, the community leadership is sympathetic to common man's needs, and the future is dependable.[4]

6. *Hypothesis V: Areas of Satisfaction in Life and Contraception*

Satisfaction in six selected areas of life was not significantly related with SES. Neither was it related with contraception. The mean score of areas of satisfaction (ASL) for the subjects of "high" SES was 3.86 ($SD = 1.36$), and the corresponding mean for the subjects of "low" SES was 3.32 ($SD = 1.66$; $t = 1.57$; $df = 153$; $p > .05$). Table 2.IV shows the mean scores of ASL by early and late acceptance of contraception. The difference between the early and the late acceptors is not significant at the .05 level. The data thus indicated that when the six areas are combined, the degree of satisfaction is not related with either contraception or SES. However, contraception was related to satisfaction with the chances of old age security, achievement of short-term and long-term material goals.[5]

The data supported the first four hypotheses of this study and thus suggested that contraception is significantly and positively related with level of striving, future orientation, value orientations, and social optimism. Degree of satisfaction in all six areas of life chosen in this study was not related with

---

[4] See footnote 1.
[5] See footnote 1.

contraception. The number of living children was significantly and inversely related with contraception, but when parity was controled, the first four hypothses were substantiated. Religion was another variable significantly related with contraception. But when religion was controled, among the non-Catholics the first four hypotheses were supported. The number of the Catholic subjects was rather small for any statistical test of hypotheses. However, a significantly higher proportion of the Catholics (68.8 percent) than the non-Catholics (52.0 percent, $\chi^2 = 3.87$, $df = 1$, $p < .05$) were late acceptors of contraception.

The multiple correlation coefficient of contraception with eight independent variables (past LOS, present LOS, future LOS, FO, VO, SO, ASL, and SES) was .78 ($p < .01$; $df = 146$). Among the independent variables, present level of striving was the best predictor of contraception which alone accounted for 40 percent variances of contraception. Other top ranking predictors were socioeconomic status and future orientation.

Occupational and educational aspirations for sons, subjective class identification, and preference for a smaller family were significantly and positively related with contraception. On a dichotomous choice between subjectively defined "too many" and "too few" children, a significantly higher proportion of the early acceptors (66.6 percent) than the late acceptors (41.2 percent; $\chi^2 = 9.45$, $df = 1$, $p < .005$) chose to have "too few" children. The early acceptors were also less frequently willing to "tolerate" one or two additional children than what they considered desirable.

The use of various contraceptive methods were in the following order: oral pills (35.9 percent), diaphragm (23.9 percent), IUD (9.4 percent), condom (8.7 percent), spermicidals (7.4 percent), female sterilization (6.3 percent), male sterilization (4.8 percent), and nonappliance methods (3.6 percent). A significantly higher proportion of the early (72.4 percent) than the late (48.8 percent) acceptors felt that their contraception practices so far have been very effective or effective ($\chi^2 = 9.46$, $df = 2$, $p < .01$). Interestingly, over one-half of the subjects with one accidental pregnancy held themselves responsible for contraceptive failure, while nearly two-thirds of those with multiple accidental pregnancies, directly or indirectly blamed the contraceptive method used by them.

D. Summary

This exploratory study tests five hypotheses which predicated significant and positive relationships between contraception and following social-psychological variables: (a) level of striving, (b) future orientation, (c) value orientations, (*d*) social optimism, and (*e*) areas of statisfaction in life. These relationships were tested while socioeconomic status (SES) was held constant. The data supported the first four hypotheses of this study. Although SES was significantly related with contraception, as well as with the psychological variables, while SES was held constant, the relationships between contraception and the first four psychological variables were significant and positive. These relationships are, therefore, independent beyond the SES of the subjects.

Among the non-Catholics, the first four hypotheses were substantiated. The number of the Catholics was too small for hypotheses testing. Although parity was inversely related with contraception, when the number of living children was controled, the first four hypotheses were supported. The multiple correlation coefficient between contraception and eight independent variables was .78; the leading predictors of the variances of contraceptions are in the following order: level of striving, future orientation, and socioeconomic status.

The early and the late acceptors of contraception varied in their subjective ranking of the hopes for the future, but they were more alike in their worries for the future. The early acceptors assigned higher priorities to children's college education, long-term goals, and self-improvement goals. The late acceptors assigned higher priorities to material, short-term, and economic goals. The leading worries for both groups were related to health, economic status, children, and war or violence.

Contraception was also significantly and positively related with educational and occupational aspirations for sons, and subjective class identification. It was inversely related with the number of pregnancies and desired family size.

REFERENCES

1. CANTRIL, H. Patterns of Human Concerns. New Brunswick, N. J.: Rutgers Univ. Press, 1965.
2. CANTRIL, H., & FREE, A. Hopes and fears for self and country: The self-anchoring striving scale in cross-cultural research," *Amer. Behav. Sci.,* 1962, **6**, 2.
3. DAVIS, K. Population. *Sci. Amer.,* 1963, **209**(3), 63-71.
4. DAY, L. H., & DAY, T. Too Many Children. Boston, Mass.: Houghton Mifflin, Riverside Press, 1964.
5. FREEDMAN, R., WHELPTON, P. K., & CAMPBELL, A. A. Family Planning Sterility, and Population Growth. New York: McGraw-Hill, 1959.
6. GRABILL, W. H., KISER, C. V., & WHELPTON, P. K. The Fertility of American Women. New York: Wiley, 1958.
7. HOLLINGSHEAD, A. B. Two factor index of social position. Mimeographed paper, New Haven, Connecticut, 1957.
8. ———. Two factor index of social position. Mimeographed paper, New Haven, Yale Station, Connecticut, 1965.
9. HOLLINGSHEAD, A. B., & REDLICH, F. C. Social Class and Mental Illness. New York: Wiley, 1958.

10. KAR, S. B. Individual aspirations as related to acceptance of family planning. Doctoral dissertation, University of California, Berkeley, 1966.

11. KISER, C. V., *Ed*. Research in Family Planning. Princeton, N. J.: Princeton Univ. Press, 1962.

12. KISER, C. V., & WHELPTON, P. K. "Resume" of Indianapolis study of social psychological factors affecting fertility. Population Stud., 1953, **7**.

13. ————. Social Psychological Factors Affecting Fertility (XXXIII Summary of Chief Findings and Implications for Future Studies. New York: Milbank Memorial Fund, 1958.

14. KLUCKHOHN, F. R. Dominant and variant value orientations. In Kluckhohn, C. (Ed.), *Personality in Nature, Society, and Culture*. New York: Knopf, 1956.

15. KNUTSON, A. L. Personal security as related to station in life. *Psychol. Monog.*, 1952, **66**, 4.

16. LEWIN, K. Field Theory in Social Sciences: Selected Theoretical Papers (Cartwright, D. *Ed*.). New York: Harper & Row, 1951.

17. LEWIN, K., *et al*. Level of aspiration. In McV Hunt, J. (Ed.), *Handbook of Personality and Behavior Disorder* (Vol. I). New York: Ronald Press, 1944.

18. OSBORN, F. Qualitative aspects of population control: Eugenics and euthenics. In Shimm, M. G. (Ed.), *Population Control*. New York: Oceania, 1961.

19. RAINWATER, L. And the Poor Get Children. Chicago, Ill.: Quadrangle Books, 1960.

20. ROSEN, B. C. The achievement syndrome. *Amer. Soc. Rev.*, 1956, **21**, 203-211.

21. ROSEN, B. C., & D'ANDRADE, R. G. The psychological origin of achievement motivation. *Sociometry*, 1959, **22**, 185-218.

22. SROLE, L. Social integration and certain corollaries: An exploratory study. *Amer. Soc. Rev.*, 1956, **21**, 709-716.

23. TIETZE, C. *Ed*. Bibliography of Fertility Control: 1950-1965. New York: Nat. Committee Maternal Health, 1965.

24. WESTOFF, C. F., *et al*. Family Growth in Metropolitan America. Princeton, N. J.: Princeton Univ. Press, 1961.

KEY-WORD TITLE INDEX

AUTHOR INDEX